An Unnatural History of Emerging Infections

An Unnatural History of Emerging Infections

RON BARRETT AND
GEORGE J. ARMELAGOS

OXFORD
UNIVERSITY PRESS

An Unnatural History of Emerging Infections. First Edition. Ron Barrett and George J. Armelagos
© Ron Barrett and George J. Armelagos 2013. Published 2013 by Oxford University Press.

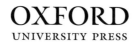

OXFORD

UNIVERSITY PRESS

Great Clarendon Street, Oxford, OX2 6DP,
United Kingdom

Oxford University Press is a department of the University of Oxford.
It furthers the University's objective of excellence in research, scholarship,
and education by publishing worldwide. Oxford is a registered trade mark of
Oxford University Press in the UK and in certain other countries

First Edition published in 2013
Impression: 1

Published in the United States of America by Oxford University Press
198 Madison Avenue, New York, NY 10016, United States of America

British Library Cataloguing in Publication Data

Data available

Library of Congress Control Number: 2013936271

ISBN 978-0-19-960829-4

Printed and bound by
CPI Group (UK) Ltd, Croydon, CR0 4YY

George: To Jack and Mary Kelso

Ron: To the ancestors, the Panchdevi, and Mike the Chimpanzee

Acknowledgements

This book is a culmination of many years of work with many people. In particular, we would like to thank Chris Kuzawa and Thom McDade, who were our co-authors on the seminal article for this book. Credit also goes to James Lin for independently noting that the current emerging disease trends represent a Third Epidemiological Transition. Thanks to Kristin Harper, who contributed to our later thinking about these transitions. Thanks to all the students in our emerging infections courses for their many questions and insights. Thanks as well to Dennis Van Gerven, Alan Swedlund, Richard Meindl, Merrill Singer, Peter Brown, Steve Hackenberger, Joe Lorenz, Ian Buvit, Brad Belbas, Erik Davis, David Woolsey, Gabe Sibley, and John and Audrey Eyler. Special thanks to Scott Legge, Christy Hansen, and Steve Sundby for their thoughts and comments on earlier drafts. Thanks to Clark Larson, Dennis VanGerven, Dan Bailey, and Gwen Robbins Schug for permitting us to use their images in this book. Special thanks to Justin Gibbens for his brilliantly provocative cover art. Ron would like to thank his colleagues at Macalester Anthropology: Dianna Dean, Margo Dickinson, Olga Gonzalez, Arjun Guneratne, Scott Legge, Sonia Patton, and Dianna Shandy, as well as his family, Ron Sr., Dianne, Tara, Maya, Tiffany, Avena, Nic, and Taiya. And a very special thanks to Lene Pedersen, Ron's colleague, partner, and writing coach, who carefully read and edited every draft of this book. And finally, we would like to thank our editors and supporters at Oxford University Press: Ian Sherman, Helen Eaton, Lucy Nash, Muhammad Ridwaan, and G. Hari Kumar for shepherding this project to completion.

Contents

Introduction

We ask the God of Plague: "Where are you bound?"
Paper barges aflame and candlelight illuminate the sky.

Farewell to the God of Plague. *Mao Zedong (1958)*[1]

Microbes are the ultimate critics of modernity.[2] Devoid of thought and culture, they can nevertheless adapt to our latest technologies by the simple means of genetic mutation and rapid reproduction. Bacteria, viruses, and other microparasites have evolved to operate in almost any human environment: in our ovens and refrigerators, in our heating vents and air-conditioning ducts. Some thrive in the industrial excrement of our oil spills, car mufflers, and smoke-stacks. Others thrive in the human body itself. No matter how many personal hygiene products we use, there will always be ten times the number of bacterial cells than human cells in our bodies.[3] Even within the human cells, we find that 8 per cent of our DNA is composed of sequences from ancient viral infections (Ryan 2004).[4] Despite our reigning civilizations, it is the microbes, not the humans, who are the colonial masters of the living world.

Outnumbered and outgunned, we should not be surprised at our inability to control pathogens, the particular subset of microbes that contribute to infectious disease. Yet for many years, this unfortunate reality did not prevent authorities from making optimistic pronouncements about the imminent demise of human infections. Sir Macfarlane Burnet, the pioneering Australian virologist and Nobel laureate, famously described the middle of the 20th century as "the end of one of the most important social revolutions in history, the virtual

---

[1] Mao Zedong was inspired to write this poem after reading a newspaper announcement that schistosomiasis had been eradicated from Yukiang Valley.

[2] For the purposes of this book, we use the term "microbe" (a contraction of "microbiological organism") in the more expanded sense to include viruses and prions as well as other microscopic parasites. Some authors exclude these entities insofar as viruses and prions do not engage in their own reproduction or metabolism.

[3] There are approximately 10^{13} human cells and 10^{14} bacterial cells in a human adult body. Yet because they are much smaller, the total biomass of these bacterial cells is a mere kilogram.

[4] These are known as Human Endogenous Retroviral sequences (HERVs). Most HERVs are "junk" sequences that no longer code for functional genes. That said, a few active HERV genes have been identified that contribute to the cellular regulation of important human tissues and sometimes produce human diseases (Ruprecht et al. 2008).

An Unnatural History of Emerging Infections. First Edition. Ron Barrett and George J. Armelagos
© Ron Barrett and George J. Armelagos 2013. Published 2013 by Oxford University Press.

elimination of the infectious diseases as a significant factor in social life" (Burnet 1962: iii). As president of the American Association of Medical Colleges, Robert Petersdorf predicted that there would be scant role for infectious disease specialists in the next century, unless, as he wrote, they would "spend their time culturing one another" (Petersdorf 1986: 478). Such statements reflected a clinical consensus that most major human infections would be eradicated by the beginning of the 21st century, and that attention and resources would be focused on eliminating the so-called chronic "diseases of civilization" such as cancer, diabetes, and heart disease. Many health policies shifted accordingly, as did funding for the prevention and control of infectious diseases.

Odds notwithstanding, the medical community had reasons to be optimistic. Infectious diseases had been declining steadily in the affluent world since the beginning of the Industrial Revolution, and similar trends could be seen in many developing nations after the end of the Second World War (Riley 2005). By 1980, smallpox had been completely eradicated from the human race. The success of this program was a major inspiration for efforts toward the global eradication of malaria, polio, tuberculosis, and other major infections (Henderson 1980). After penicillin, new antibiotic molecules had been discovered every decade up until the 1970s (Amyes 2001). The revolutionary new field of molecular biology promised even smarter medicines informed by the genetic sequences of disease causing microbes and their human hosts. In the face of these developments, one might understandably conclude that pathogens were on the eve of extinction.

Yet while medical leaders were dissuading would-be infectious disease specialists, the AIDS pandemic was already well underway. The AIDS virus was among more than eighty newly identified human pathogens discovered between 1980 and 2005, including Legionella, Ebola, Marburg, and highly pathogenic strains of *V. cholera* and *E. coli* (Woolhouse and Gaunt 2007). International support for major disease eradication programs had declined, as had domestic support for public health programs aimed at the prevention and control of infections among the poorest segments of the richest nations. In developing nations, an ever-growing division between rich and poor impeded recent gains in infectious-disease mortality (Armelagos et al. 2005). With global poverty as a reservoir, infections once thought to be under control returned instead to cross borders and haunt the affluent as "re-emerging" diseases. Tuberculosis (TB) was a prime example of this re-emergence. Long considered a receding plague of poverty, TB returned to the world's wealthiest nations with a vengeance (Farmer 1997). Moreover, it did so at time when these wealthy nations were experiencing their first increases in infectious-disease mortality after more than a century of decline (Jones et al. 2008).

Worse still, these new and recurring diseases demonstrated increasing resistance to antimicrobial drugs. Since the early days of penicillin, bacteria had been steadily evolving resistance to antibiotics within a few years of their development and use (Normark and Normark 2002). Although researchers continued to develop newer drugs, these substances were no more than clever modifications of less than two dozen truly unique, core molecules. Even at the time of this publication, no new core molecules have been discovered since 1961 (Amyes 2001). Meanwhile, an increasing number of serious infections, tuberculosis among them, were showing resistance to more than one type of drug (Kim et al. 2005). It appeared that the rates of microbial evolution had outpaced the technological revolutions of their human hosts, and that we were rapidly moving toward a post-antibiotic era: a time when we would no longer have the medicines to safely cure bacterial infections.

With increasing awareness of these developments, optimism turned to concern in the 1990s. During this time, health professionals coined the phrase "emerging and re-emerging infections" to describe significant increases in new, recurring, and drug-resistant diseases. The phrase was echoed in the titles of several conferences, a major publication by the Institute of Medicine, and an academic journal produced by the US Centers for Disease Control and Prevention (Lederburg et al. 1992; Satcher 1995). These projects pointed to factors of globalization and shortcomings in public health policies and programs. They also shared a common purpose of increasing public awareness, spurring new research, and rekindling previously neglected health initiatives. But unlike the medical optimists of the previous decades, their main objective was considerably less ambitious.

It is unrealistic to expect that humankind will win a complete victory over the multitude of existing microbial diseases, or over those that will emerge in the future. . . Still, there are many steps that scientists, educators, public health officials, policymakers, and others can and should be taking to improve our odds in this ongoing struggle. With diligence and concerted action at many levels, the threats posed by infectious diseases can be, if not eliminated, at least significantly moderated.

(Lederburg et al. 1992: 32)

By framing the problem as one of emerging and re-emerging infections, the medical community succeeded in raising public awareness about a global health issue, but important lessons were misunderstood or lost in translation. Despite good intentions, fear got the better of reason as the concept of emerging infections spread to the popular media. Films such as *Outbreak* and best-selling books such as *The Hot Zone* focused public attention on a few novel diseases with putative origins in exotic foreign lands (Preston 1994). They cast gruesome images of people bleeding from all orifices and rotting to death, while emphasizing that, in this interconnected world, any infection was only a plane flight away (See Figures 0.1a and 0.1b). Perhaps more damaging, these stories promoted high-tech and military-style interventions, over basic public-health measures, as the most effective approach for controlling these diseases. Unfortunately, the military approach was popular among policy-makers as well, even more so after the anthrax attacks of 2001, when resources for preventing known disease threats were diverted to biosecurity programs aimed at threats such as smallpox (Cohen et al. 2004; Barrett 2006a).

However well intended, the terms "emerging" and "re-emerging" are prone to misunderstanding, especially when they convey a false sense that the problem of human infections is new, or that their appearance is sudden and spontaneous. Neither is the case. To begin with, not all newly identified pathogens are actually new to human populations—HIV and legionella being two prominent examples. Physicians first became aware of AIDS in 1981 when an unusually large number of patients appeared in US hospitals with either a rare form of cancer or a pneumonia not often found in younger adults (Centers for Disease Control and Prevention 1981). Researchers identified HIV a few years later and developed a test for the

(a)

(b)

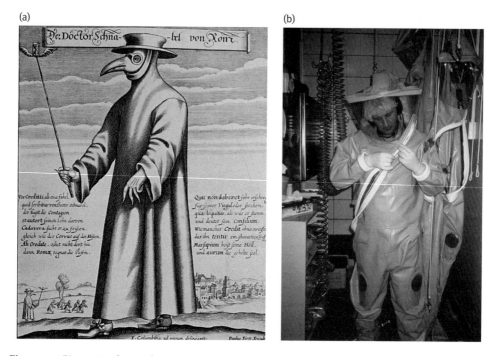

Figure 0.1. Biosecurity then and now. The illustration on the left is an engraved copper plate of a 17th-entury plague doctor wearing a protective suit. The beaked mask contained materials designed to filter out "bad air." The contemporary photograph on the right is a technician donning a positive-pressure biohazard suit before entering one of the US Centers for Disease Control's (CDCs) maximum containment laboratories. While conveying safety concerns, such images can also spread unnecessary alarm, stigmatize populations, and distort public perceptions of risk. Engraving from Eugen Hollander 1921. *Die Karikatur und Satir in der Medizin.* Stuttgart: Ferdinand Enke. Photograph by Brian Mahy, Centers for Disease Control and Prevention.

virus. Building on this knowledge, researchers then tested preserved blood samples from patients who had died of similar opportunistic diseases, revealing HIV infections going back to 1959 (Zhu et al. 1998). Similarly, after Legionnaire's disease made its debut at an American Bicentennial convention, retrospective studies of preserved tissue samples revealed that the *Legionella* bacterium was responsible for at least 2000 deaths that had been previously diagnosed as nonspecific pneumonias (Meyer 1983). Because of examples like these, epidemiologists are often careful to use the phrase "newly *identified* pathogen" rather than "new pathogen" when describing novel infections.

Furthermore, the term "re-emerging infections" is only relevant for diseases previously assumed to be under control, assumptions usually made in affluent societies that have long since benefited from declining infectious disease rates. The phrase makes little sense in poor societies where the same infections had never declined in the first place. For example, smallpox had declined for two centuries in Western Europe and North America until it became a rare disease after the Second World War, but the infection nevertheless persisted in underdeveloped nations, particularly in South Asia and sub-Saharan Africa. With the permeability of national borders and social boundaries, smallpox periodically (and predictably) returned to the affluent West in the form of fifty-three limited outbreaks over the next thirty years before its final eradication (Barrett 2006a). These outbreaks were known as re-importation epidemics. Today they would be known as re-emerging infections.

Given these considerations, when does an infection qualify as an emerging or re-emerging infection? Some public health workers joke that it is when the first white person contracts it. Cynical though this may be, the joke reflects a global situation in which pathogens are freely transmitted between nations and societies, but the solutions to these infections are often segregated and contained (Farmer 1996). As such, wealthy societies are sometimes able to deny attention and sufficient resources to certain diseases; that is, until they make a surprise return to the developed world. Such is the situation today, which is notable less for emerging pathogens themselves and more for an emerging human awareness of long-standing problems that never went away.

With the aim of emerging awareness, this book examines the human determinants of infectious diseases from evolutionary, historical, and critical social perspectives. The current spate of human infections is certainly a major global problem, and some of these diseases are indeed new to our species. However, the underlying determinants of these problems are anything but new. Our susceptibility to infectious diseases is primarily the result of human activity patterns spanning human history and prehistory. These patterns involve changing modes of subsistence, environmental disruptions, population shifts, and social inequalities. While the pathogens themselves are a natural and ever-present feature of our environment, the conditions in which they evolve are highly unnatural insofar as they are shaped by deliberate human actions, however unintended the consequences of these actions may be. Such infections are the artifacts of human culture and their history is essentially an *unnatural* history.

Epidemiologic Transitions

The current phenomenon of emerging and re-emerging infections is the result of shifting health and population patterns known as epidemiological transitions (Barrett et al. 1998). Currently, we are experiencing the latest of three major epidemiological transitions that occurred between the Neolithic and the present day. The First Transition was linked to a major shift in human lifestyles from nomadic foraging to a more sedentary lifestyle and the beginnings of agriculture around 10 000 years ago (Armelagos and Harper 2009). The Second Transition was linked to the Industrial Revolution beginning in Western Europe and North America in the 18th century, and continuing in different forms among some developing societies after the Second World War. The Third Transition is marked by the accelerated globalization, urbanization, and aging associated with the so-called emerging and re-emerging infectious diseases of today (Barrett et al. 1998).

Abdel Omran first introduced the concept of the epidemiological transition as a theoretical model to explain how changing disease patterns affected major population changes associated with the Industrial Revolution (Omran 1971). This model was built on a Demographic Transition Model that population scientists had previously used to describe the shift from high birth and death rates (fertility and mortality, respectively) to low birth and death rates in wealthier nations undergoing industrial economic development (Caldwell 1976). This was an important observation, but the Demographic Transition Model simply pointed to associations between economic and population changes; it did not address their underlying causes. Omran sought to address this shortcoming by showing how the changing epidemiology of major diseases affected population change. His goal was to focus attention "on the complex change in patterns of health and disease and on the interactions between these patterns and the demographic, economic, and sociological determinants and consequences" (Omran 1971: 510). It was an ambitious attempt to bring together experts from different disciplines to understand the underlying determinants of a major shift in the health and demographic patterns of large human populations.

To demonstrate his model, Omran collected historical population data from as many countries as he could. However, because the wealthier countries had more complete and reliable data, he mainly focused on Europe and North America in what is often referred to as the Western or Classic Transition Model. With less data, Omran also formulated a Delayed Transition Model for underdeveloped countries undergoing more recent and modest forms of this transition. We will return to the Delayed Model when we address the issue of re-emerging infections in later chapters. For now, we will focus on the better-known Classic Model.

Omran divided the Classic Epidemiological Transition into three stages, the first of which he called *The Age of Pestilence and Famine*. This age was characterized by populations in which high fertility rates were offset by high mortality rates—families gave birth to many children, but many of these children also died from infectious diseases and under-nutrition. For instance, in 17th-century Sweden, a country now known for its excellent health statistics, birth rates ranged from 5–10 per family, but at least a third of these infants died before the age of one, and half the remaining children did not survive to adulthood (McKeown 1988). These days, it would be difficult for any parent with reasonable means to imagine the loss of even a single child, let alone the deaths of three children or more. But for many centuries, this was a common experience in state-level societies around the world. One could easily characterize this period as "the bad old days."

Following this tragic baseline, Omran described an *Age of Receding Pandemics*, beginning in Western Europe around the middle of the 18th century. In this period, countries began to experience modest declines in the endemic, or day-to-day infections, that had been typically present in their populations. More importantly, they also experienced significant declines in the frequency of unusually large epidemics or pandemics, such as the smallpox, plague, and typhus outbreaks that sporadically appeared every few decades and swept away millions of lives in their wake. These changes brought an increase in life expectancy to about 40–50 years of age. Of course, major infectious epidemics did not recede altogether. The industrial world continued to experience major disease events. Overall levels of endemic infections remained quite high as well, but with a noticeable leveling of the disease spikes that characterized centuries past. If we were to liken infection to a body of water, one could say that the seas were calmer, even if overall water levels were high compared to the present day.

The Age of Degenerative and Manmade Diseases is the third and final stage of Omran's Classic Epidemiological Transition. This brought major overall declines in infectious disease mortality from the late 19th to mid-20th-centuries. Life expectancy increased dramatically during this period, as much as thirty years in many countries. But life expectancy is a special kind of average that can be easily misinterpreted. In this case, increased life expectancy did not mean that adults were living to older ages so much as children were surviving to adulthood, primarily because of declining infections. In place of these infections, chronic degenerative diseases such as cancer and heart disease became the major causes of death in the industrialized world. This Classic Transition was largely responsible for the optimism in the 1960s and 1970s regarding the future demise of human infections (see Figure 0.2).

Omran's theory has been criticized for its emphasis on unilinear and universal change, its selective focus on the health of white males, and its assumption that industrial development is the primary engine for health and demographic change (Salomon and Murray 2002). We share these concerns, but would rather address them in more fundamental terms and with an eye toward improving the model. As Omran intended, the Classic Transition does help to explain complex interactions between economics, demographics, and disease rates, but the model has two important shortcomings. The first is historical: the concept of a single epidemiological transition suggests that pre-industrial societies have always suffered from high rates of infectious diseases, which is not the case. For the majority of our evolutionary history, human beings lived in small nomadic forging groups, lifestyles that were not conducive to the spread of acute and virulent infections. It was only after we began settling down and domesticating

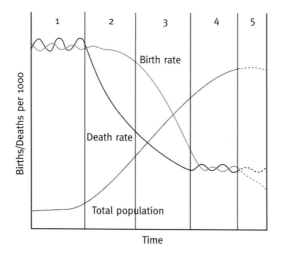

Figure 0.2. Mortality decline resulted in overall population increases in affluent nations around the time of the Industrial Revolution, despite declining fertility rates. While demographic transition theorists described this phenomenon earlier, Omran's classic epidemiological transition specifically linked these changes to declining infectious diseases. Creative Commons Public Domain.

plants and animals that infectious diseases became a major human problem—this was actually our first major epidemiological transition.

Even with recognition of delayed transitions in developing nations, the second major shortcoming of Omran's model is that it primarily addresses economic changes in affluent societies, implying that developing societies will experience similar changes once they have become sufficiently modernized. Although many poorer societies underwent some degree of transition in the decades following the Second World War, these declines were more modest than in their affluent counterparts, and more dependent on antimicrobial medications facing an increasing threat of drug-resistant infections (Riley 2005). At the same time, these countries were experiencing the challenges of aging populations and chronic degenerative diseases, a situation that could be characterized as the worst of both worlds.

Far from a single, universal, or unilinear event, these epidemiological transitions have arisen in various forms and trajectories in different societies and historical periods. Yet with the rapid globalization of these different societies, humankind is now converging into a single disease ecology, one that involves a convergence of disease patterns as well as the transmission of pathogens across populations and national boundaries. This convergence represents a Third Epidemiological Transition, characterized by the accelerated evolution of human transmissibility, increased virulence, and drug resistance among infectious pathogens. Globalization notwithstanding, the underlying determinants of this latest transition are much the same as the first. Although industrial technologies have accelerated and expanded these problems, the same human activities have shaped and reshaped the evolution of human infections for the last 10 000 years.

Organization of this Book

Our unnatural history begins in Chapter 1 with the prehistoric baseline preceding the first major rise of acute infectious diseases in the human species. This baseline consists of nomadic foraging lifestyles and their health implications during 99.995 per cent of our evolutionary history. While there is much debate about the particulars of these lifestyles and the supporting evidence, there is general agreement that the basic parameters of nomadic foraging could not sustain the kinds of acute and highly virulent infections that we see today. Such diseases require large, densely populated, and highly interconnected populations for sustained transmission. Transmission of acute infections would not have been possible in the small and sparsely distributed groups that characterized the social organization of our nomadic ancestors.

Nutritional states are closely linked to disease susceptibility, and we know from studies of contemporary foragers that hunting and gathering leads to richly varied diets high in lean protein and fiber, and low in unhealthy cholesterols and fat. While foraging societies may have dealt with seasonal shortages and lower overall caloric intake, they were less likely to experience the micronutrient deficiencies that would compromise immunity and increase susceptibility to the infections that we see in their agricultural counterparts. Additionally, foraging does not entail prolonged contact with animals, an important factor when we consider that the ancestry of many human infections can be traced to strains that were originally adapted to domesticated animals. Finally, it should be noted that while known foraging societies are by no means free of conflict and cruelty, they do not display the degree of social hierarchy and inequalities that are commonly seen in state-level societies, populations where the destitute often serve as points of entry and reservoirs for infection.

In Chapter 2, we apply the tools of bioarchaeology to examine ancient societies undergoing the transition from nomadic foraging to sedentism and agriculture. Comparing the health states of human remains before and after this transition, we find that the foraging groups were significantly healthier than their agricultural descendants. This evidence—situated in the context of dense populations, poor diets, animal-borne diseases, and social inequalities—strongly supports the theory that the Agricultural Revolution resulted in diminished nutritional status and higher infectious-disease mortality for human populations around the world. These were the first truly emerging infections in the human species.

Agriculture begat the First Epidemiological Transition, characterized by a major rise in acute infectious diseases, which would persist at high levels in densely settled societies of the Old World until the 18th century. Human populations increased as well, displacing foraging societies and transforming the lands around them. Indeed, such increases were necessary to meet the demands of labor and military forces. But they also came at the terrible cost of high childhood mortality for diseases like smallpox, plague, yellow fever, and malaria that would become endemic to the Eurasian continent. These and other food and water-borne infections would later sweep Native-American populations following the Columbian invasions of the New World. Enabled and perhaps exceeded by human violence, these New World pandemics were the tragic consequence of sudden contact between pre- and post-transition societies.

Moving on to the Industrial Revolution, Chapter 3 examines the decline of infectious diseases in affluent nations of Europe and North America from the 18th–20th centuries. This Second Transition gave rise to the medical optimism in the decades prior to the so-called emerging and re-emerging infections of today. Much of this optimism was based on a strong belief in the efficacy of modern medicine, as well as its theories and technological advancements. Yet in contrast to these beliefs, the development of Germ Theory had little to do with the Second Epidemiological Transition in industrialized societies. Furthermore, with the exception of smallpox vaccination, infectious diseases underwent most of their declines before the advent of effective antimicrobial medicines. Rather than new medical theories and technologies, the determining factors of declining infections were improved nutrition and living conditions, and better distribution of these essentials across social groups. Although scholars debate the relative contributions of particular factors, few disagree with the primary role of changing lifestyles in this transition. Viewed from a much deeper time line, we could say that the lifestyle factors associated with this Second Transition—those concerning subsistence, settlement, and social organization—were essentially improved versions of those that instigated the emerging infections of the First Transition thousands of years earlier.

Chapter 4 examines the Second Transition in developing societies from a critical perspective that helps explains today's so called re-emerging infections. In the years following the Second World War, many poorer nations experienced declining rates of infectious-disease mortality. These declines, however, were more modest than those experienced by their wealthier neighbors. They were also closely linked to the use of antimicrobial medicines, a troubling issue given the recent rise of multi-drug-resistant infections. At the same time, the developing world experienced the same rising rates of chronic degenerative diseases associated with the Second Transition in well-developed countries, a "worst-of-both-worlds" syndrome (Bradley 1993).

At this point, we introduce the concept of syndemics: interactions between multiple diseases that exacerbate the negative effects of one or more disease (Singer and Claire 2003). Syndemics include co-infections, the best-known examples being AIDS-related infections such as tuberculosis, cytomegalovirus, and cryptococcal meningitis. Less well-known but very prevalent are co-infections of influenza and bacterial pneumonias; the latter are actually the primary cause of flu-related deaths (Sethi 2002). Chronic respiratory diseases such as asthma and emphysema increase susceptibility to influenza and other respiratory infections; there is also a strong association between diabetes and tuberculosis. If we include the effects of social diseases—violence, substance abuse, malnutrition, and so forth—then we could easily argue that syndemics constitute the vast the majority of re-emerging infections.

With syndemics in mind, we must consider that the First and Second Epidemiological Transitions did not proceed one from the other in direct, linear progression, nor were they universally experienced or even fully complete. Moreover, the accelerated globalization of human societies and their diseases are bringing these incomplete trends into collision, resulting in a Third Epidemiological Transition characterized by the entry of new pathogens to the human species, and the evolution of virulence and antimicrobial resistance in long-standing diseases. The remaining chapters of this book are dedicated to examining these phenomena.

Chapter 5 applies very old lessons to newly identified or newly virulent diseases. Given that the majority of these infections are evolutionary descendants of zoonotic (i.e. animal borne) infections, we consider the manner and conditions required for the entry and sustained transmission of these pathogens within our species. Here, we re-encounter the same major themes of the Neolithic—changing patterns of subsistence, settlement, and social organization—but with more complex tools and larger, faster moving populations. Commercial agriculture has driven marginalized groups into previously uninhabited environments, where practices such as bushmeat hunting have increased the risk of blood-borne infections from wild animals, including those apes most closely related to us, and other nonhuman primates (Wolfe et al. 2005). Commercial agriculture has also increased the size and density of domesticated animals (and their stress levels) such that they are more likely to incubate zoonotic diseases and pass them on to humans (Davis 2006).

In the early stages of contact with humans, zoonotic infections often exhibit "viral chatter" in which a zoonotic pathogen evolves the ability to "jump" to human hosts, but not yet to the degree that it can sustain further transmission in human populations (Wolfe et al. 2005). The resulting "chatter" is a set of sporadic and limited outbreaks among people engaged in certain high-risk activities. Such was the case during recent outbreaks of pathogenic avian influenza, in which the majority of infected people were people engaged in commercial poultry activities, but with no further spread to immediate contacts (Dinh et al. 2006). Repeated incidents like these increase the risk that a new pathogen will evolve the ability for human-to-human transmission. However, even human-to-human transmission may not be sustainable, depending on conditions such as the density of the host population and their overall susceptibility to diseases.

Unfortunately, conditions for the sustained transmission of new human infections are rich and plentiful. The majority of the human race now resides in dense, urban environments, and the majority of these urban residents live in poverty (Dye 2008). Urbanization is often associated with decreased fertility, which in turn leads to increasing proportions of elderly over time. This aging of human populations is not only occurring in affluent nations, but also in developing nations with fewer resources to care for them (Kinsella and Velkoff 2001). Consider that the immune systems of these poor, aging, and densely settled populations are further compromised by food insecurity, industrial pollution, and diminished access to clean water and sanitation, as well as associated pneumonias, parasites, and diarrheal diseases. Include mosquitoes, substance abuse, and high-risk sexual practices in the mix, and then consider how globalization has connected these populations within a day's travel with everyone else in the world. Accounting for all these conditions, we must conclude that our present world is a fertile field for the germination and proliferation of new infections.

Many of these conditions are also ripe for the evolution of drug resistance in human and animal pathogens. Chapter 6 explores whether this evolution will inevitably lead to a post-antimicrobial era. To better understand the problem, we first examine the pre-human evolution of antibiotics as natural defenses of microorganisms in competition with one another. We also consider evidence for the use of antibiotic substances, such as the tetracyclines, in ancient and traditional healing practices prior to, or aside from, those informed by Germ Theory. Without a concept of microorganisms, we can reasonably infer that these practices were focused on patient characteristics and those of their surrounding environments. This was certainly the case for the sanitary reform movements of the 19th century. Although mistaken about the microscopic causes of human infections, the sanitarians had very good ideas about host susceptibility, disease-prone environments, and effective methods of addressing these factors to prevent and control the spread of disease.

The sanitary approach changed little during the early years of Germ Theory, which initially produced more academic discoveries than effective biomedicines. During this period, the metaphor of "soil and seed" was regularly invoked by biomedical physicians who increasingly believed in Germ Theory but continued to practise environmental medicine: just as the growth of crops requires the right characteristics of both soil and seed, so the growth of infections requires the right characteristics of both environment and pathogen. Not much could be done about most pathogens until the middle of the 20th century, so the focus was on internal and external environments: good nutrition, exercise, clean surroundings, and isolation measures that minimized contact with other people and animals—an apt prescription for Paleolithic living.

The clinical focus changed with the growing concept of "magic bullet" medicines that could target pathogens, like military snipers, while leaving the host unharmed. The magic bullet concept began with the bacterial selectivity of dye compounds and gained momentum with the development of Salvarsan (also known as arsphenamine, or Compound 606) for the treatment of syphilis (Amyes 2001; Winau et al. 2004). Applying evolutionary theory to bacterial competition, biochemists discovered many antibiotic substances in soils and sewers around the world and developed them into pharmaceuticals. But in many cases, drug-insensitive and drug-resistant infections began to appear within a few years after the adoption of a new antibiotic. In an effort to counter these developments, chemists would either search for new molecules, or alter the original molecules into the next generation of drugs. Bacteria would then develop resistance to these new drugs, and so on. In this way, the magic bullet concept expanded to an arms race concept, with growing concerns that humans are losing the race (Sachs 2007).

Returning to the prospect of a post-antibiotic era, we note with some irony that the mechanisms of antibiotic resistance, like the antibiotics themselves, are natural products of microbial competition that evolved prior to human interference (D'Costa et al. 2011). We then examine major ways that humans have accelerated the evolution of drug resistance, beginning with the overuse and misuse of these drugs around the world. But as with most health practices, the solutions are not simple matters of education and behavior change. We must consider the economies of time and money for patients and their healers alike. Second, we turn to the role of commercial agricultural practices, which include the use of antibiotics as animal growth factors. Third, we reconsider the role of syndemics with respect to susceptible host populations that provide reservoirs for incubation at the early stages of drug resistance (Barrett 2010). Finally, we examine evidence for the persistence of drug resistance despite local changes in drug use (Andersson and Hughes 2011). Given these data, it may be that resistance is inevitable, yet this may not be the worst scenario when we recall that our modes of living have had far greater impact on the prevention and control of infectious diseases than all our pharmaceuticals combined.

There was a time when a "social disease" referred only to a sexually transmitted infection (Morrow 1904), but the recurring theme of this book is that all human infections are essentially social diseases. With this in mind, we conclude our unnatural history with a discussion of how the social lessons of three epidemiological transitions can be applied to improving the prevention and control of infectious diseases. The most important improvement would be to re-organize our approach to these problems. Most health institutions are organized vertically, such that their attention and resources are divided according to certain diseases rather than their underlying determinants. Yet if the same determinants can be found in nearly all these diseases, then a horizontal approach would be more effective—one that addresses how we feed ourselves, how we live in relation to our social and natural environments, and how we distribute basic resources for our health and well being. This approach must also cross national and social boundaries because now that we live in a global disease ecology, the health of anyone can affect the health of everyone.

Part One

The First Transition

1

The Prehistoric Baseline

…humans living today are Stone Age hunter-gatherers displaced through time to a world that differs from that for which our genetic constitution was selected.

Stone agers in the fast lane. Eaton et al. (1988a: 739)

Scholars have long held opposing views about our earliest human ancestors, the nomadic foragers who wandered the world for more than a hundred millennia prior to the advent of agriculture, writing systems, and state-level societies. In *The Leviathan*, Thomas Hobbes argued for a centralized state which would prevent the negative consequences of humanity's earliest and most "natural" form of social organization. With this agenda in mind, Hobbes described our ancient ancestors as living in "continual fear and danger of violent death," an existence which he infamously summarized as "…solitary, poor, nasty, brutish, and short" (Hobbes 1651: XIII.9). A century later, Jean Jacques Rousseau issued a strong rebuttal in his *Discourse on Inequality*, asserting that "natural man" was free and living in "celestial and majestic simplicity, as created by the 'divine Author'" (Rousseau 1754: 6). Shaped by political philosophy more than empirical evidence, neither of these extreme views carried much scientific validity.

Even with the evidence against them, the ghosts of Hobbes and Rousseau continue to haunt more recent anthropological debates about ancient and contemporary foraging societies, comprised of people often known as hunter–gatherers. Some describe them collectively as the "original affluent society" based on observations of egalitarianism and lighter workloads among certain living groups (Sahlins 1968). Others paint a bleaker picture, pointing to archaeological and ethnographic evidence of violence, food shortages, and gender inequality (Kaplan 2000). As in most academic debates, the answer probably lies somewhere between the extremes, and as with most human issues, the answer is probably subject to considerable variation.

We hold an intermediate position on the topic, one that is based on a modest interpretation of the evidence and an acknowledgement of human cultural variation. Within these parameters, we argue that certain basic patterns of subsistence, settlement, and social organization were widely shared among ancient foraging societies. More importantly, we argue that these patterns precluded exposure and susceptibility to the kinds of acute infections that have been observed in agricultural societies from the earliest farmers 10 000 years ago to the global industrialized cities of today.

An Unnatural History of Emerging Infections. First Edition. Ron Barrett and George J. Armelagos
© Ron Barrett and George J. Armelagos 2013. Published 2013 by Oxford University Press.

These prehistoric living patterns hold several important keys to the understanding and prevention of acute infectious diseases. First, they illustrate how certain modes of subsistence produced the dietary diversity needed to build immunity against pathogens. Second, they illustrate how modes of settlement can affect the widespread transmission of infections based on the geographic dispersal of host populations. Finally, these patterns illustrate how social organization can affect potential reservoirs of infection based on the distribution of essential resources. The foraging lifestyle was not a panacea against all diseases; hunter–gatherers faced challenges of parasitic infections, seasonal food shortages, and exposure to natural toxins. But we can safely argue that ancient hunter–gatherers did not experience the severity and frequency of acute infections as did the agriculturalists who followed them. It is important to understand the reasons for these differences, because the same factors affect our risk for acute infections today, albeit at faster speeds and much larger scales.

Our prehistory also provides evolutionary insights into why our species is susceptible to certain diseases. It could be said that modern day humans are "stone agers living in the fast lane" (Eaton et al. 1988a). Despite our technological advancements, the pace of human biological evolution has been so slow that our bodies have changed little since *Homo sapiens* first appeared in the Middle Paleolithic around 100 000 years ago. If a Paleolithic person were to appear today dressed in a business suit, he or she would easily blend in with the variety of people we would expect to find at an international airport or train station. In cultural terms, our lifestyles have radically changed since the Paleolithic, with billions of people living in urban environments, moving about in machines, and shopping for industrial foods in globally connected markets. Yet in biological terms, we are little different from our prehistoric ancestors who once hunted barefoot on the African savanna.

The mismatch between our cultural and biological makeup has important implications for our susceptibility to new, recurring, and drug-resistant infections. To begin with, our risk of contracting infectious diseases is closely linked to the global burden of chronic, non-infectious diseases such as diabetes, heart disease, and many forms of cancer. Tuberculosis (TB) is much more prevalent among people with adult onset diabetes, and in some places, this risk is comparable to the risk of TB among people with HIV/AIDS in the same populations (Ponce-De-Leon et al. 2004). Diabetes and heart disease have been associated with higher mortality among people infected with the SARS virus, as well as to those infected with highly pathogenic strains of influenza (Chan et al. 2003). Such examples are known as syndemics, defined as the interaction between two or more epidemic diseases so as to magnify the negative effects of one or both diseases (Singer and Clair 2003). In many cases, chronic diseases become syndemic with infectious diseases by suppressing the immune system and putting sick people in close contact with each other via frequent and lengthy hospital stays. Both factors combine to produce a large reservoir of susceptible hosts, especially for pathogens that are just beginning to infect human populations.

Thinking in terms of prevention, many of us understand that chronic diseases are strongly linked to our modern modes of living: our diets, our activities (or lack thereof), and the modified environments around us. Professionals and pundits tell us *how* these so-called "lifestyle factors" are bad for our health. They tell us that how cholesterol-rich diets can lead to heart disease through the accumulation of plaques in our arterial walls. They tell us how, for many of us, an excess of processed sugars can lead to adult onset diabetes by overwhelming our ability to metabolize glucose. They also tell us how physical exercise helps us maintain optimum blood pressure and overall weight. But while we may understand the *hows* of healthy living, few of us understand *why* certain lifestyles are better or worse for human health.

To answer this quandary, we must recognize that our present-day lifestyles are very different from those in which we evolved. Anthropologists refer to these earlier lifestyles as our environments of evolutionary adaptation (EEAs). Our EEAs hold the keys to human health. For about 90 000 years, biologically "modern" humans lived as nomadic foragers on the savannas and grassy woodlands of Africa and the temperate zones of Europe and Asia. Prior to this, our prehuman (i.e. hominid) ancestors lived under similar conditions for another 4 million years. This adds up to 99.995 per cent of our evolutionary history in which the human body had genetically adapted to a nomadic foraging lifestyle (see Figure 1.1). It would take more than a thousand generations for our bodies to catch up with the cultural changes that occurred in the barest fraction of the time that our species and its forbears have been on this planet. In the meantime, we must contend with the hazards of calorie-rich diets, physical inactivity, and exposure to industrial pollution. Not surprisingly, popular health messages for avoiding these hazards are essentially prescriptions for living more like our Paleolithic ancestors (Eaton et al. 1988b).

Given these health implications, it is important that we examine our prehistoric baseline: the EEAs of nomadic foraging societies that prevailed until the time we first settled down and domesticated our food sources around 10 000 years ago. Despite some methodological challenges, we can identify basic and common themes about how these people lived in terms of their diet and activity patterns, their relationships with other species, and their demographics and social organization. These same themes will recur throughout this book as we explore the three epidemiological transitions leading to the global health challenges of the present day. Then as now, these social and cultural themes comprise the "unnatural" determinants of emerging infectious diseases.

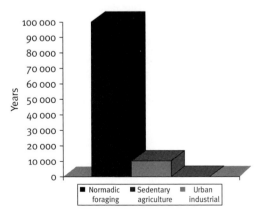

Figure 1.1. Histogram comparing number of years that humans spent engaged in nomadic foraging, sedentary agriculture, and urban industrial modes of living.

1.1 Nomadic Foraging: Then and Now

Our understanding of Paleolithic living is based on two major lines of evidence: archaeological remnants of ancient foragers, and ethnographies of contemporary hunter-gatherer societies whose conditions are reasonably analogous to those of the past. For the archaeologist, the Paleolithic presents several challenges for data collection. First, there were not many people around back then, so there were not many human remains to dig up. At the height of the Paleolithic, there were only about 8 million people living in the world, a little over a thousandth of the total human population today (Coale 1974; Bloom et al. 2011).

Second, there is the challenge of finding the few remaining bodies. It would have been impractical for nomadic societies to dispose of their dead in common locations. Such practices would require that people carry heavy, decomposing corpses across long distances. It was far more efficient to dispose of corpses near the places where people died, which would have also been places near where people lived—i.e. scattered across great distances. This pattern of scattering is supported by the archaeological record, which reveals few instances of collective, ceremonial burials before the end of the Paleolithic and no actual cemeteries until the Neolithic (Munro and Grosman 2010).[1]

Third, there is the challenge that these small, nomadic societies did not leave much stuff around. They left no written records and had no more possessions than they could carry on their backs. They also tended to build structures that lasted for seasons rather than generations. In contrast, current societies are leaving behind mountains of garbage for future archaeologists. The United States alone produces 160 million tons of garbage a year, with 15 per cent of its foodstuffs going directly into the trash (Lilienfeld and Rathje 1998). Perhaps more than our libraries and museums, this discarded waste will say a great deal about our industrial lifestyles. Not so with Paleolithic foragers, who possessed little and wasted even less.

Despite these methodological challenges, there is still sufficient evidence to determine some basic but important characteristics of our Paleolithic ancestors. Although they did not leave many artifacts behind, ancient foragers left remnants of their daily diets in cooking hearths and trash pits known as middens. These sites contain the charred and butchered bones of wild as opposed to domestic, animals indicating that they obtained their meat through hunting rather than husbandry (Wiener and Wilkinson 2011). In addition, the minute

---

[1] Although there is some evidence suggestive of ceremonial burials dating from the Middle Paleolithic period, it has also been noted that natural post-mortem (i.e. taphonomic) processes can mimic intentional burial (Gargett 1999). The most famous examples are the Neanderthal burials of Shanidar Cave, where pollen found with the bodies suggested the use of flowers (Solecki 1971: 102). Later evidence suggests the pollen was the result of rodent activity (Sommer 1999). The earliest clear-cut evidence of ceremonial burial has been found at Hilazon Cave in Israel, where feasting on wild cattle and tortoises occurred around 12,000 BP (Munro and Grosman 2010).

particles of plant material left behind at these sites provide a rich source of data. There is an entire sub-field of archaeology, known as palynology, that examines the particular character-istics of these ancient pollens, spores, and other tiny organic particles. By examining the mor-phology and genetics of these particles, palynologists confirm that the flora associated with known Paleolithic sites were wild as opposed to domestic varieties (Salamini et al. 2002). Similar evidence has been found in ancient human fecal remains, known as coprolites (Speller et al. 2010). All told, this evidence confirms that, until about 10 000 years ago, human beings obtained their food by hunting wild animals and gathering wild vegetation. There may have been some small-scale horticulture, as we see in many contemporary foraging societies, but not of the duration and scale to produce detectable environmental changes.

The hunting and gathering lifestyle is not conducive to large and densely clustered human populations. In the African savannas where the earliest humans lived, current hunter–gatherers require an average of about one square mile per person to obtain an adequate diet from their local environment. Such spacing requires that human beings live in small, widely scattered groups, a principle supported by the archaeological record. With the exception of ancient coastal fishing communities, most archaeological discoveries reveal human groupings of no more than thirty to forty people (Kelly 1995; Binford 2001; Marlowe, 2005). In order to maintain these small groups, ancient foragers must have either maintained zero population growth for very long periods of time, somehow balancing their birth rates with their death rates, or else they must have dealt with increasing population through subsequent group divisions and migration to other territories (Pennington 2001). We should note, however, that although these strategies may have persisted for a very long period of time, they were not without problems. Indeed, such problems may have eventually driven humans to systematic agriculture.

In addition to human artifacts, there is also a great deal to be learned about the health of Paleolithic foragers from their skeletons and teeth. We will examine this evidence in the next chapter when we compare the overall health of societies before and after the transition from foraging to agriculture. In the meantime, we can take this basic information about subsist-ence and demography and examine contemporary foraging societies as analogous examples of Paleolithic living. But as with the archaeological data, these ethnographic data present a number of unique challenges. One such challenge is environmental and cultural representa-tion. All human societies were foraging just before the Neolithic, but societies who are cur-rently engaged in this lifestyle represent less than 0.001 per cent of the human population today (Pennington 2001). As such, we might regard contemporary foragers to be exceptional cases, especially when we consider that many of their local environments are in remote or inhospitable locations, places that are impractical for modern settlement.

Among today's remaining foraging societies, none could be considered pristine in the sense of being untouched by the industrialized world or even living continuously in the same manner. The well-studied !Kung San bushmen of the southern African Kalahari had experi-mented with pastoralism long before they met their first anthropologist (Lee 1990). The Punan of Borneo probably shifted from agriculture to foraging in order to trade forest products with the Chinese (Hoffman 1986), and contemporary Martu women of Western Australia prefer to use LED headlamps for hunting at night and iPods for listening to Lady Gaga (Bird Personal

Communication 2010). These shifting patterns and cultural contacts have sparked debate among anthropologists about the extent to which contemporary foragers are culturally representative of our prehistoric ancestors (Ames 2004; Guenther 2007).

Yet even when we recognize these limitations, there are basic characteristics of subsistence, population structure, and social organization for which contemporary foraging societies may serve as models for Paleolithic living. These societies provide a wealth of ethnographic and ecological data as well as insights into the disease patterns of our nomadic foraging ancestors. Here, diversity works in our favor, for if we find that these basic characteristics are shared across different cultures and environments, then these ethnographic findings provide even stronger support for our thesis. Supplementing these findings with bioarchaeological data, we can then begin to reconstruct our prehistoric "disease-scape."

1.2 Subsistence, Nutrition, and Activity

Closely tied to human immunity, nutrition has always been our chief line of defense against infectious diseases. Conversely, malnutrition is the chief determinant of immunosuppression worldwide (Chandra 1997). The human immune system demands a significant amount of metabolic energy, if only to defend ourselves from the daily pathogens we encounter under the best conditions. These demands increase further under worse conditions. During a severe infection, the immune system needs immediate glucose, stored in the form of glycogen, to produce and mobilize antigen-specific cells, immunoglobulins, and other signaling molecules. The body initially meets these demands by becoming hyperglycemic until its glycogen stores are depleted (Ullrey 2005). After this, the body catabolizes the proteins of muscle cells, converting its constituent amino acid acids into additional glucose.

In addition to glucose, protein energy is essential for immune function. Protein energy malnutrition is associated with decreased antibody production, thymus and lymph node reduction, and diminished function of phagocytes, cytokines, and t-lymphocytes (Smith et al. 2005). Studies have found that people with protein deficiencies who were less than 85 per cent of their expected body mass for size were comparable to AIDS patients regarding their compromised cell-mediated immune function (Schaible and Kaufman 2007). Micronutrients also play important roles. Iron-deficiency anemia has widespread impact throughout the immune system. Zinc deficiency is associated with the breakdown of cell membranes at critical areas of pathogen entry such as the skin, pulmonary mucosa, and gastrointestinal tract; vitamin A deficiency is similarly associated with the breakdown of tissue barriers at potential entry points for infection (Field et al. 2002). The human body needs more than calories to have a properly functioning immune system; it must meet a broader range of nutritional requirements. Prior to industrial food production, dietary diversity was the only way to achieve this nutritional breadth.

From tropical to temperate environments, most contemporary foragers have highly diverse diets in comparison with agriculturalists in the same regions; they are even more diverse than some industrialized societies (Cordain 2002). This diversity is well illustrated in the !Kung San of the southern African Kalahari desert, who regularly hunt thirty-four different species of animals, and occasionally hunt another twenty-four species (Lee 1990). The San identify fourteen edible fruits and nuts, fifteen edible berries, forty-one roots and bulbs, and another seventeen vegetables that a westerner might find in his or her salad (Lee 1990). Prior to settlement, the Ache of Paraguay hunted fifty-six animal species and gathered another forty-four plant species as well as honey (Hill and Hurtado 1996: 74). Studies of the Australian Anbarra, the East African Hadza, and the Central African Efe reveal similarly diverse diets (Jenike 2001).[2] The diversity of these diets increases the likelihood of meeting all nutritional requirements for health in general, and healthy immunity in particular. Thus, we should not be surprised to find evidence that our species has evolved physiological "incentives" for seeking a variety of foods (Rolls et al. 1982; Ó Gráda 2009).

Dietary breadth also has several other important advantages. Chief among them is behavioral flexibility in the face of changing environmental conditions. Droughts, floods, and crop diseases can have a devastating impact on societies that depend on only a few food types for their subsistence. We have seen this with the Irish Potato Famine of the 18th century as well as the Ethiopian and Chinese famines during the latter half of the 19th century (Ó Gráda 2009). Although these events were influenced by important political and socio-economic factors, their impact was greatly exacerbated by reliance on only one or a few different food sources. Societies that can obtain a variety of foods under different conditions are buffered against the potential hazards of these environmental crises, especially when they can resort to a range of "famine foods" during severe shortages. Finally, the ability to forage a variety of foods allows greater migratory flexibility for nomadic groups that may need to travel through relatively scarce regions to arrive at more plentiful destinations (Hawkes and O'Connell 1992).

In addition to having broad and balanced diets, foragers commonly eat foods that are high in protein, high in fiber, and low in saturated fats. Meat from wild animals is much leaner than from domestic varieties, and carbohydrates are found in vegetables rather than processed grains. Combining the bioarchaeological evidence with data from contemporary foragers, it is estimated that most Paleolithic foragers consumed six times the fiber of the average American today, and that the latter consumes almost twice the calories from dietary fat (Eaton and Eaton 2000). Biometric studies of societies that engage almost exclusively in foraging typically find that members are thinner and have higher aerobic capacities than those in industrial societies (Cordain et al. 2000). Consequently, these people also have lower rates of diabetes, heart disease, and several forms of cancer (Eaton et al.1994; Eaton et al. 1988a; Eaton and Eaton 2000).[3]

With these data in mind, two physician-anthropologists heralded the merits of diets that are nutritionally similar to those of our Paleolithic ancestors in the *New England Journal of Medicine* (Eaton and Konner 1985). These recommendations were expanded in *The Paleolithic Prescription* (Eaton et al. 1988b). Other authors followed with less rigorous science and flashier titles such as

[2] It should be noted that there is less dietary diversity among arctic foraging societies with much higher ratios of animal protein. That said, these diets usually cover all essential nutrients and are less prone to unforeseen shortages than among their temperate and tropical counterparts (Kelly 1995).

[3] The opposite case can be found among highly acculturated ex-foragers, which often have unusually high rates of diabetes and cardiovascular disease, leading some to propose a Thrifty Gene Hypothesis in which such populations would have greater sensitivity to insulin as a biological adaptation to previously leaner diets (Yajnik 2004; Neel 1982).

Neanderthin and *Charley Hunt's Diet Evolution* (Audette and Gilchrist 1995; Hunt and Hunt 2000). Subtitles reinforced the case: "Eat Like a Caveman to Achieve a Long Lean Body," and "Get Healthy Eating the Food You Were Designed to Eat" (Audetteand Gilchrist 1995; Cordain 2002). But with all this interest in ancient eating, it could be said that most safe and sensible diets are at least as similar to a Paleolithic diet as they are to one another. The Paleolithic prescription is perhaps best summarized in Michael Pollan's popular phrase, "Eat food. Not too much. Mostly plants." However, for the sake of authenticity, one may wish to add wild game to the list.

Along with these significant benefits, there are also drawbacks to a Paleolithic-style foraging diet. To be a reliably successful forager requires considerable skill and experience, to include a detailed knowledge of plants, animal behavior, tracking, navigation, and weather patterns. Hunting and gathering usually requires significant energy investments. An adult !Kung San woman, who is typically twice as efficient at obtaining food as her male hunting counterparts, expends an average 2500 calories over two hours gathering 23 000 calories-worth of food (Lee 1990). Compare this with the modern suburban shopper, who may expend 100 calories over the 20 minutes it takes to obtain the same 23 000 calories. Of course, this does not count the effort needed to earn the money for the food, which could range from 150–400 calories an hour, depending on whether the shopper sits at a desk or performs heavier tasks in an urban environment. Yet even by conservative estimates, the !Kung San forager expends about seven times more energy than the shopper to extract the same amount of calories.[4]

Foraging also involves a great deal of uncertainty. Although most foragers have a broad range of food sources to choose from in their environments, they may face seasonal shortages of edible plants and wild game, forcing them to range over longer distances in search of better opportunities (Hawkes and O'Connell 1992). Large-game hunting entails physical risks in the pursuit and killing of animals, including the risk of falling prey to other carnivorous animals. Even consuming plant foods may entail significant risks; many wild food staples contain high percentages of cyanide-like substances and other toxins specifically harmful to the liver, gut, and central nervous system (Johns 1996). Government-approved industrial foods may not always be as nutritious, or even "food" per se, but they rarely pose the same risks for poisoning as raw plants found in the wild.

Lastly, foraging diets also pose a greater risk of exposure to parasites. Foragers in the Paleolithic were probably afflicted by two classes of parasites known as heirloom species and souvenir species (Kliks 1990; Sprent 1969). Heirloom parasites refer to species that we inherited from our pre-human (i.e. hominid) ancestors insofar as they continued to infect them as they evolved into modern humans. Most of us are well acquainted with heirloom parasites, having at some point experienced pinworms or head and body lice (see Figure 2). They also include internal parasites such as *Salmonella typhi*, and certain kinds of staphylococci (Cockburn 1967; Cockburn 1971).

The souvenir parasites are those "picked up" by foragers as they carried out their daily activities. Most of these parasites were zoonotic, meaning that their primary hosts were nonhuman animals that only incidentally infected humans through contact such as insect

---

[4] These kinds of comparisons support Marshall Sahlins' famous assertion that hunter–gatherers represent the original affluent society (1968).

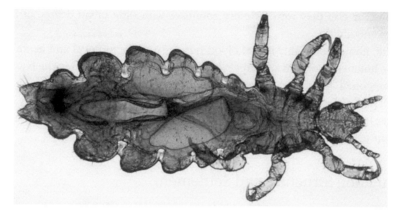

Figure 1.2. Photograph of a female head louse (*Pediculus humanus var. capitis*). Head lice were probably heirlooms that we inherited from our nonhuman primate ancestors. Following the Neolithic, lice would become vectors of more acute and virulent diseases such as typhus. Photograph by Dennis Juranek, Centers for Disease Control and Prevention.

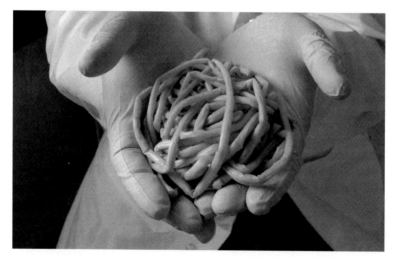

Figure 1.3. Mass of Ascaris lumbricoides worms that had been passed by a child in Kenya. Humans first acquired these kinds of helminth (i.e., worm) infections during ancient migrations into new environments. Ascaris is typically transmitted in egg-form via fecal-oral route. Photograph by James Gathany. Provided by Henry Bishop, Centers for Disease Control and Prevention.

bites, animal bites, contact with animal urine and feces, and the preparation and consumption of contaminated flesh. These souvenir parasites included trypanosomiasis (also known as sleeping sickness), tetanus, scrub typhus, relapsing fever, trichinosis, avian or ichthyic tuberculosis, leptospirosis, schistosomiasis, and a variety of tapeworms (Cockburn 1971; Froment 2001) (see Figure 1.3). But although these parasites were probably endemic to ancient hunter–gatherers, most existed as chronic infections that people could live with and carry around, or else they were primary zoonoses with little or no degree of human-to-human transmissibility.

Paleolithic hunters probably risked blood-borne exposure to novel and acute infections through the butchering of wild animals. We will examine this issue later in the book when we examine the potential role of contemporary bushmeat hunting for the entry of new viruses into human populations (Wolfe et al. 2005). But unlike today's large and globally connected populations, Paleolithic hunter–gatherers lived in small, scattered groups that could not have sustained the acute, human-to-human infections that we see today.

1.3 Population Structure and Settlement

Acute infections require large and dense host populations to sustain themselves. Measles is a prime example of this principle. A medieval descendant of the bovine rinderpest, the measles virus is so contagious that 90 per cent of unvaccinated people could contract the disease simply by sharing the same room with an infected person (Furuse et al. 2010). Yet measles rarely persists in small, relatively isolated and unvaccinated populations that have been exposed to the virus. A classic study following nineteen native Caribbean island communities over fifteen years found that measles outbreaks were self-limited in unvaccinated populations of less than 500 000 people. Similar dynamics were found for measles in the Faro islands, the common cold on the Norwegian island of Spitsbergen, and poliomyelitis among isolated communities of northern Native Alaskans (Black 1980).

This is not to say that small, insular populations are free of viruses. Another study found many isolated native Amazonian groups with antibody titers for herpes and Epstein-Barr viruses that were comparable to suburban populations in the eastern United States (Black 1975). The key here is that herpes and Epstein-Barr often persist as chronic, recurring infections in human hosts. Like the heirloom and souvenir parasites of Paleolithic foragers, chronic viruses can be carried for long periods of time and thus do not require frequent transmission in order to maintain themselves in human populations. In contrast, a highly contagious disease with rapid onset, such as measles, may spread rapidly in a small group—often with devastating effects—only to extinguish itself before it can be passed on to other groups.

Even in more socially connected societies, a viral epidemic can extinguish itself if the onset and course of the disease is too rapid and severe to allow a sustainable rate of transmission among potential human hosts. Such is the case for Ebola hemorrhagic fever. From 1976–2009, there have been seventeen outbreaks of the disease in central African nations ranging from the Ivory Coast to the Sudan (CDC 2011). These outbreaks were severe, with mortality rates between 37 and 100 per cent among known victims; yet all of them ended with no more than a few hundred victims, even in the absence of vaccines or curative treatments.[5] Such numbers are unacceptable nonetheless, but it is worth noting that this terrible virus did not spread

---

[5] At the time of this publication, several potential vaccines are being developed for Ebola and similar filoviruses (Geisbert et al. 2010).

in the manner of many other pandemic diseases such as AIDS, TB, or malaria. Indeed, it is probably because of its terrible nature that the spread of Ebola has thus far been self-limited. Like HIV, the Ebola virus is primarily transmitted through blood and body fluids.[6] But unlike HIV, Ebola incubates in days rather than years, producing severe and recognizable symptoms during the period of infectivity. Consequently, the disease tends to "flash out" in human populations.

Consider these transmission principles in the context of foraging populations. The largest cross-cultural sample of contemporary foragers consists of 478 different societies around the world (Marlowe 2005). This sample is primarily based on the Human Relations Area Files, a massive database of ethnographic studies conducted by anthropologists over the course of many decades. Within the total sample of foragers, the median local group size is thirty people, usually comprising a few family units in a band or camp. There is still considerable group-size variation, especially when fishing communities in northern temperate zones are included. However, the median group size further decreases to twenty-five people in a sub-sample of 175 non-equestrian, warm-weather foraging societies—groups living in conditions more akin to those of the late Paleolithic, far smaller than the island and Amazonian societies in the epidemiologic studies above. It seems unlikely that acute infections such as measles, influenza, or smallpox could sustain themselves in societies consisting of such small groups.

That said, we should still account for rates of social mobility between these local groups. With high enough rates of inter-group exchange, some foraging societies might approximate the conditions of larger populations, at least in terms of disease transmission. Ethnographic studies often reveal a great deal of social fluidity within these groups, with families and subgroups breaking off and reforming because of shifting opportunities, interpersonal conflicts, or changes in adult sex ratios (Kelly 1995). But these fission–fusion dynamics occur over the course of months and years, far longer than the incubation periods of most major human infections. Furthermore, the overall population densities of foraging societies are very low. In the warm-climate sample above, the median local group area is 175 square kilometers, with a median overall population density of less than one person per five square kilometers (Marlowe 2005). We could reasonably expect that Paleolithic densities were at least as low, if not lower, given the much smaller total human population at the time. With this kind of dispersion, inter-group contact would be infrequent—so too would be the opportunities for inter-group infection.

In addition, the geographic mobility of foraging societies serves to minimize environmental exposure to potential pathogens. Foragers in the cross-cultural sample move an average of seven times per year (Marlowe 2005). Such mobility is important for tracking the movements of animal prey, taking advantage of seasonal changes in resource opportunities, and avoiding resource shortages as well as the total depletion of local areas. Depending on the ecological variation of the migratory region, mobility can also reduce the amount of time spent in a

---

[6] There are some reports of potential air-borne transmission, but only in cases where patients vomited or coughed blood in very close proximity to care-givers (Dowell et al. 1999).

given micro-environment, where certain zoonotic pathogens might otherwise evolve the ability to infect human hosts over time. We will return to this issue in later chapters when we examine the evolutionary dynamics of new and drug-resistant pathogens.

Lastly, the mobility of hunter–gatherers reduces the accumulation of materials that could serve as vectors of infection. Waste inevitably accumulates, even in the best-maintained camps. Burying feces and food waste outside the perimeter would still attract insects and animals to the area. Food stores and cooking areas would be attractive within the perimeter and closer to human hosts. The size of these stores may increase with the length of residence, and longer durations of storage increase the risk of the food itself becoming contaminated. Likewise for the size and duration of water storage and the probability of contamination by pathogens or insect vectors. Changing locations, even on a seasonal basis, would significantly reduce these accumulations and their concomitant risk of infection.

1.4 Social Organization and Inequalities

In the introductory chapter, we discussed the epidemiological problem posed by socio-economic inequalities in a globally connected world. If political borders and social boundaries are permeable to pathogens, but impermeable to preventive resources, then the higher risk of infection among those with fewer resources will result in increased and ongoing risks for everyone else. We see this in diseases that could have been eradicated long ago, such as poliomyelitis, which still persists in impoverished communities from South Asia to sub-Saharan Africa. In addition to the avoidable cost in lives, the risk posed by these endemic areas results in US$1.5 billion per year of direct vaccine costs worldwide (Ehreth 2003). Poverty can also serve as an incubator for new and resistant disease strains, such as Multi-Drug-Resistant and Extremely Drug-Resistant Tuberculosis (MDR-TB and XDR-TB). The highest incidences of these deadly infections have been found thus far among refugee, slum, and prison communities around the world (Kim et al. 2005; Wright et al. 2009). Yet it is unlikely that new TB strains will contain themselves to these so-called "hot spots." We should therefore regard impoverished communities as vulnerable points of entry for new infections in a globally connected population.

Long before globalization, the inequality principle would have still applied to insular foraging societies of the Paleolithic. The dispersion of nomadic foragers may have prevented sustained transmission of acute and highly virulent pathogens, but not so for parasites and other chronic infections. Within local groups, an equitable distribution of food resources, workload, and the care of children could have had profound effects on individual susceptibility to these latter diseases. If resource and labor distributions were greatly imbalanced, then some would be more vulnerable to initial infection, which they could eventually pass on to others. As with any socially interconnected group, the risk of infection among foraging groups would be largely determined by the disease susceptibility of their most vulnerable members.

Such inequalities are uncommon among contemporary foraging societies due to their relatively egalitarian social structures and sharing practices. Unlike the formal hierarchies of many tribal and village societies, band-level foraging groups are most often characterized by informal leadership and consensus decision-making (Lee and Daly 1999). Although hunting and gathering requires a great deal of specialized knowledge, foraging groups have little need for divisions of labor beyond those of sex and age. And perhaps most importantly, nearly all contemporary foragers display strong beliefs and practices regarding the sharing of food and other resources, despite considerable linguistic, cultural, and environmental variation (Ingold 1999; Winterhalder 2001).

Egalitarianism and sharing would have been as adaptive for Paleolithic foragers as it now is for their contemporary descendants. Formal leadership would add an unnecessary layer of complexity to small social groups, and it would not be enforceable without having consensus in the first place. Furthermore, it would also be unnecessary to divide labor specialties beyond those of basic subsistence and care-giving. Indeed, further specialization may even be hazardous, given the flexibility needed by people to exploit a variety of resources in changing environments. Sharing also allows for flexibility insofar as all members can share the risk of differential food returns for any given foraging activity. This is especially relevant when geographic mobility sets physical and temporal limits on material accumulation. Without the margins of excess accumulation, reciprocity is the best insurance against unpredictable returns.

This is not to suggest that foraging lifestyles are free of inequalities and conflicts. Many ethnographic studies reveal gender inequalities—instances of men obtaining better cuts of meat, or women doing a disproportionate share of the work (Endicott 1999; Gurven and Kaplan 2007). Some groups experience high levels of violence, which can be a significant reason for group fissions and relocations (Gurven and Kaplan 2007). Yet even when faced with these challenges, most foraging societies are far more egalitarian and equitable in their distributions and duties than their agricultural counterparts. It therefore follows that the concomitant risks and benefits for health and disease would also be more equitably distributed in local foraging groups than in agricultural communities. No single individual or subgroup would be more vulnerable than another.

1.5 Conclusion

This chapter illustrates how human lifestyles and human inequalities can mediate our susceptibility and exposure to infectious diseases. Nomadic foraging has been the dominant lifestyle of our species and its forbearers for the vast majority of time that we have been on the planet. Examining this lifestyle, we can observe links between subsistence and immunity via the dietary diversity of hunter-gatherers. We can also observe links between the dispersion and mobility of human populations and the feasibility of sustained transmission for different kinds of potential pathogens. Lastly, we see links between social organization and intra-group susceptibility based on the distribution of essential resources for healthy living.

With consideration of these factors, a picture emerges of Paleolithic foragers as neither idyllically affluent nor nasty and brutish. Somewhere between these extremes, we recognize significant challenges posed by seasonal shortages, interpersonal violence, and chronic, parasitic infections. But we can also argue that Paleolithic foragers did not experience the kinds of acute infections that we see in sedentary agricultural societies leading to the present day. That said, most of our supporting evidence thus far has been based on observations of contemporary hunter–gatherers, and the assumption that these basic-level lifestyle data are analogous to those of our Paleolithic ancestors. The next chapter will provide further confirmation when we directly examine the bioarchaeological record of ancient populations as they transitioned from a baseline of nomadic foraging to a sedentary agricultural lifestyle. We will see how this transition, sometimes known as the Agricultural Revolution, profoundly changed our relationships to the microbial environments around us—relationships that continue to the present day.

2

Revolution and the Domestication of Pathogens

…I have placed a curse on the ground. All your life you will struggle to scratch a living from it. It will grow thorns and thistles for you, though you will eat of its grains. All your life you will sweat to produce food, until your dying day.

Genesis 3:17–19

The greatest revolution since the beginning of humankind was more radical and fundamental than any single change of government, major technology, or world view. After a thousand centuries of nomadic hunting and gathering, our ancestors began settling into permanent residences and domesticating plant and animal food resources (Armelagos et al. 1991). This Agricultural Revolution transformed the planetary biosphere and ultimately fueled a thousandfold expansion of the human population. It triggered a cascade of major cultural changes, from emerging states to emerging industries. It also led to what could arguably be called our first "emerging infections:" an unprecedented increase in acute infectious diseases as the primary cause of human mortality. We define this increase as the First Epidemiologic Transition (Barrett et al. 1998).

The Agricultural Revolution did not happen all at once, nor did it spread from a single source. The earliest known evidence of its beginnings occurred between 10 000 and 8000 years BCE in the Near East between the Tigris and Euphrates Rivers, a region commonly referred to by archaeologists as the Fertile Crescent, the same region that would later see the rise of Mesopotamia and the present-day countries of the Persian Gulf (Harlan 1971; MacNeish 1992). This particular instance of domestication is famously known as the Neolithic Revolution, although genetic studies of plant and animal varieties point to additional centers and times for the independent adoption of agriculture in the Far East, Central Africa, and Central and South America (Piperno 2001).[1] From these centers, the Agricultural Revolution spread across the world over a period of 9000 years, until more than 99.99 per cent of the human population settled down and shifted to farming and animal husbandry as a primary mode of subsistence (see Figure 2.1).

---

[1] Nikolai Vavilov conducted some of the earliest research on the origins of domestication. He hypothesized that the centers of plant domestication would have the greatest variety of wild species that were closely related to the first domestic crop.

An Unnatural History of Emerging Infections. First Edition. Ron Barrett and George J. Armelagos
© Ron Barrett and George J. Armelagos 2013. Published 2013 by Oxford University Press.

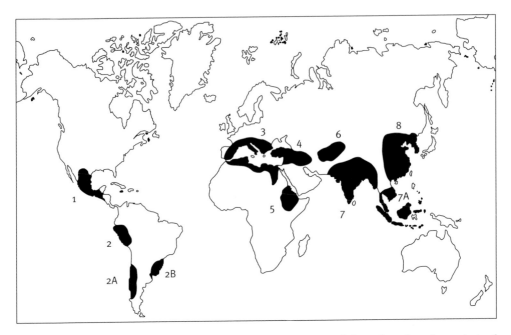

Figure 2.1. Geographic centers for the independent domestication of plants, based on the analysis of species diversity by Nikolai Vavilov. These include: (1) Mexico–Guatemala, (2) Peru–Ecuador–Bolivia, (2A) Southern Chile, (2B) Southern Brazil, (3) Mediterranean, (4) Middle East, (5) Ethiopia, (6) Central Asia, (7) Indo-Burma, (7A) Siam–Malaya–Java, (8) China. Map provided by Redwoodseed 2008. Creative Commons Attribution Share Alike 3.0.

Given the extent of the revolution, it is puzzling that human societies did not switch to farming earlier, or at least did not do so in earnest. Yet the archaeological record clearly shows that our primary reliance on plant or animal domestication probably did not begin much before 8000 BCE (Piperno 2001).[2] Some have argued that domestication never occurred to people before then, but that once people understood the connection between seed and plant, agriculture would have been the sensible and lasting choice. Others have posited that a gradual accumulation of knowledge occurred under the right environmental conditions until people saw the added value of agriculture and adopted the process as a primary means of subsistence (Braidwood 1967).

It is unlikely, however, that knowledge was a limiting factor in the adoption of agriculture. Ethnographic studies of contemporary foragers around the world underscore how successful hunting and gathering requires extensive knowledge of the biology, behavior, and life cycles of particular flora and fauna (cf. Lee 1969). Such knowledge would have been more than sufficient to begin the process of domestication. Indeed, there is evidence for the harvesting of small seeds dating back to the Upper Paleolithic, and most contemporary forag-

---

[2] The earliest evidence for plant domestication is 23 000 years old, but evidence for primary reliance on farming or husbandry does not appear until much later (Weiss et al. 2001).

ing societies engage in some degree of horticulture for secondary subsistence (Kelly 1995).[3] It was not for want of understanding that it took our species 100 000 years to adopt agriculture as a major way of life. Something else must have prompted the revolution.

Archeologists have proposed many theories to explain the origins of agriculture, most of which emphasize environmental or demographic determinants, with discoveries playing a secondary role as the process later became intensified.[4] Environmental theories point to major triggers such as climate change and droughts that desiccated foraging areas, thereby concentrating people, plants, and animals into small oases of cultivation. V. Gordon Childe famously argued that the "propinquity" of plants, animals, and humans in these oases would make domestication inevitable, since intensive interaction with certain plants and animals would lead to a greater understanding of their exploitation as food sources. In places with little evidence of environmental catastrophe, alternative theories have focused on longer-standing, oasis-like features, such as the "hilly flanks" of the mountains surrounding the Fertile Crescent and the Levant region of the Middle East (Braidwood 1983).

Demographic theories point to the destabilization and expansion of human populations, not to the degree that would later happen with the intensification of agriculture, but enough to place pressure on societies beyond their capacities for effective and peaceful foraging (Cohen 2009). The reasoning follows that, having expanded into all habitable regions of the planet, human populations first began experiencing these pressures in the late Pleistocene. Such theories explain surges of animal exploitation in places and times of sudden population expansion (Stiner et al. 1999). There are also multi-causal theories that combine environmental and demographic variables (MacNeish 1992). Yet for all these explanations, few emphasize the benefits of sedentariness and domestication, except in relation to negative events or pressures that led up to the change. The consensus is that human societies were pushed more than they were pulled into agriculture.

These revised theories do not suggest that we should return to a life of hunting and gathering, but they do raise the question as to why *Homo sapiens* adopted agriculture as a means of subsistence in the first place. We have become such "Neolithic chauvinists" that to even raise the question seems misguided. For some students of human evolution, it seems incredible that *Homo sapiens* took so long to "discover" agriculture. As we will show, there were and still are biological and social costs associated with the intensification of agriculture. There is also evidence suggesting that many foragers in Europe resisted the use of the Neolithic technology as it moved into the continent (Price and Gebauer 1995).

---

[3] Many nomadic pastoral societies have also engaged in horticulture. It should also be noted that pastoralism represents an ancient way of living that does not fit into the foraging or agriculture categories. While worthy of examination, we are omitting such studies in this book for the sake of space.

[4] There are also Marxian and cultural–materialist theories that emphasize changing modes of production in the rise of agriculture (See Cohen 2009). But these theories explain historical change rather than agriculture, which is itself a mode of production. It would be circular to propose that agriculture arose *because of* a changing mode of production.

People would not have adopted agriculture unless it offered at least some advantages. Farming domestic cereal grains allows for the concentration and storage of basic calories. Raising domesticated animals offers reliable, if not always abundant, protein returns—much like putting money in the bank for later withdrawal. Both farming and husbandry provide an abundance of food energy for large or expanding populations that, in turn, allow for the further specialization of labor. This specialization often includes dedicated armies that can either defend territory or further expand it through military conquest. Foraging societies could hardly stand up against such numbers and forces, which explains why most have been displaced, assimilated, or annihilated by the expanding reach of their agricultural neighbors.

It is notable, however, that most of these advantages are competitive. As we shall see, each has also proven to be a double-edged sword—sometimes literally so. Increased food energy from domestication often came at the expense of dietary diversity, resulting in nutritional deficiencies. Expanding populations were often necessary to meet the heavier labor demands of farming. The specialization of labor was often associated with social hierarchies and social inequalities, and wars were often fought for the sake of territory, something that has always been more a dilemma for sedentary than nomadic societies. Yet for all these problems, it would have been very difficult to turn back after a certain point due to the transformation of natural landscapes, increasing populations that relied on stored calories, and the eventual loss of knowledge and experience needed for sustainable foraging. For better and worse, the road to agriculture was usually a one-way street.

We can see how the Agricultural Revolution involved much more than domestication of plants and animals. In this chapter, we will also see how it also involved the domestication of pathogens by creating selective conditions for their evolution and spread as acute human infections. However unintended, the human activities surrounding agriculture—our subsistence practices, settlement patterns, and social organizations—created opportunities for microorganisms to make the leap from nonhuman to human hosts, and then sustain human-to-human transmission within increasingly large, dense, and susceptible host populations.

Using the tools of paleopathology, we will conduct a comparative examination of human remains from ancient societies undergoing the transition from nomadic foraging to sedentary agriculture. Here, we will see how health changes in these populations provide tragic and compelling evidence for the First Epidemiologic Transition. Turning from prehistory to history, we will see even more catastrophic examples with the European invasion of the Americas, events that brought post-transition societies of the Old World into violent collision with pre-transition societies of the New World—a major step toward the globalization of human disease ecologies.

2.1 Measuring the Health of Dead People

We can learn a great deal about the health of dead people from their bones and teeth. Barring anomalies and amputations, the human body contains 206 bones that, in addition to maintaining structure and protecting vital organs, are responsible for the production of blood cells and the maintenance of overall chemical balance throughout our lives. Even after thousands of years, these bones can display telltale "signatures" of particular diseases

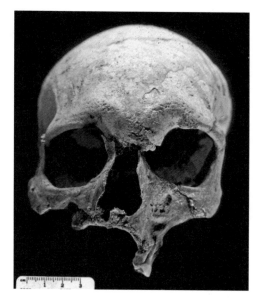

Figure 2.2. Some infections can be easily identified by certain bone deformities. These skull deformities are related to a severe form of Hansen's disease (also known as leprosy), caused by a mycobacterium that is closely related to pathogen responsible for tuberculosis. This skull is approximately 4 000 years old, originating from the Indus Valley civilization of northern India. It is considered to be the oldest likely example of this disease in the human skeletal record. Reproduced with permission of Gwen Robbins Schug.

(see Figure 2.2). Such is the case for advanced forms of tuberculosis, which can be identified by spinal decompression and the sequential breakdown and healing of bone surrounding the spinal cord and other joints throughout the body (Armelagos and Brown 2002). Other mycobacterial infections, like leprosy, and treponemal infections, like syphilis and yaws, can be identified in areas where bone tissue has been resorbed (i.e. dissolved and absorbed into the body), especially in the bones surrounding the nose and jaw (Armelagos and Baker 1988).

Bones can also reveal more general traces of bacterial infections. The invasion of gram positive bacteria, such as those of the "staph" and "strep" varieties, can affect the fibrous outer membrane of the bone known as the periosteum. Inflammation beneath this fibrous layer causes tiny hemorrhages that stretch the periosteum and produce a visibly roughened appearance (see Figure 2.3). These periosteal reactions can be observed centuries after death, although such data should be verified by triangulation with other kinds of evidence (Armelagos and Brown 2002). Triangulation is essential in any case, not only for verifying particular observations, but also for inferring all the events that we cannot observe. For every detectable pathogen, there are many more microorganisms, including most viruses, that can cause severe illness and even death without ever leaving a trace on a remaining skeleton. To infer these infections, we must use every available method to situate any potential disease events within larger contexts of health and living.

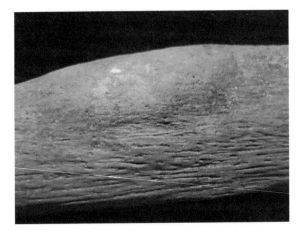

Figure 2.3. Periosteal reaction, clearly visible by the roughed appearance on this femur. Periosteal reactions are commonly associated with gram positive bacterial infections. Reproduced with permission of Dennis Van Gerven.

Nutrition and physical development provide important contexts insofar as they are closely linked to human immunity and host susceptibility. As with certain infections, there are also several nutritional diseases that leave telltale signatures. These include rickets, caused by a deficiency of vitamin D, which is essential to calcium metabolism. Rickets affects bone density and cortical thickness, resulting in a characteristic bowing of the femur (Mays et al. 2006). Scurvy is a vitamin C deficiency, once infamous among sailors on long voyages, that can produce certain tooth defects when acquired in childhood, although these are more difficult to detect in prehistoric populations (Stuart-Macadam 1989). Iron deficiency anemia is perhaps the most detectable of specific nutritional deficiencies, recognized by porous, coral-like lesions on the flat bones of the skull and the roof of the eye orbits. These lesions, known as porotic hyperostoses, result from the body's excess production of red blood cells in the bone— a physiological attempt to acquire more iron in the blood. This excess production expands the porous inner layer of trabecular bone, and exposes it after thinning the smooth outer layer until it disappears (see Figure 2.4). While anemia can also be caused by genetic conditions, like sickle cell and beta thalassemia, the relative degree of hyperostosis on the skull and its presence in small children are strong indicators of long-term iron deficiency in the diet, and a potential response to systemic infections (Wapler et al. 2004).

Teeth are often the best-preserved specimens in the skeletal record, and they provide some of the best evidence about ancient nutritional states. Dental caries (cavities) and dental-wear patterns can provide direct clues as to particular kinds of diets, such as the intake of processed carbohydrates or the proportions of soft and hard foods. These data can be triangulated with elemental bone analyses, in which certain isotopic ratios can indicate the degree of animal protein consumed, and whether it was primarily obtained from marine or land animals (Reitsema et al. 2012; Armelagos and Brown 2002).

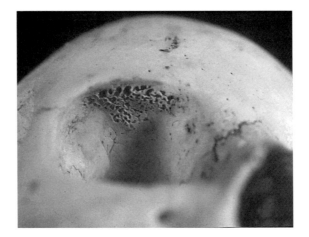

Figure 2.4. A special form of porotic hyperostosis known as cribra orbitalia, seen in flat bones of the inner eye orbit. Porotic hyperostoses are typically caused by long-term anemia which, in turn, increases susceptibility to infectious diseases. Reproduced with permission of Dennis Van Gerven.

Our knowledge of enamel development during childhood provides even more telling evidence. A growing body secretes and deposits tooth enamel in sequential layers over time, much like the rings on a tree. Like tree trunks, cross-sections of tooth crowns provide a chronological record of health states during critical periods of development. Relative rates of enamel formation result in layers of different thickness—thicker layers represent relatively healthy periods, and thinner layers (known as hypoplasias) represent relatively unhealthy periods, when development is interrupted or delayed by malnutrition, infection, or other major stressors (Armelagos and Harper 2009) (see Figure 2.5).[5] With these methods, framed within the context of other archaeological data, we can begin to measure the health of ancient populations. More importantly, perhaps, we can compare these measurements between populations living under different conditions.

2.2 Societies in Transition

The best evidence for the health impact of sedentism and agriculture comes from bioarchaeological studies of societies undergoing this lifestyle transition. Using the tools of paleopathology, we can track health changes associated with changes in subsistence, settlement,

---

[5] Enamel hypoplasias can also be caused by genetic defects or trauma. But defects are not as frequent as infections, and trauma does not produce the kinds of widespread hypoplasias that appear in children suffering from systemic diseases or other health problems (Armelagos et al. 1991).

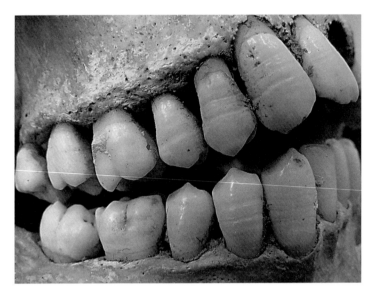

Figure 2.5. Linear enamel hypoplasias revealing periods of physiological stress, such as malnutrition or infectious diseases, during critical periods of development. Photograph by Rebecca Watts.

and social organization. Because these changes occurred within the same populations, we can rule out the possibility that differences in disease susceptibility were due to genetic variation between groups. Moreover, because these data have been uncovered in different geographic regions and historical eras, we can also rule out the possibility that they were due to common initial conditions in their surrounding natural and cultural environments. Left with our remaining variables of interest, we can focus on the net impact of the Agricultural Revolution on human health in general, and on human infections in particular.

Bioarchaeological studies yield significant evidence for health changes with agriculture in at least a dozen transitional societies in Asia, Africa, Europe, and North and South America (Cohen and Armelagos 1984). With few exceptions, the health outcomes for agriculture are poor in these studies. Near the Fertile Crescent, excavations in Iran and Iraq reveal higher rates of child mortality from the Late Paleolithic to the Neolithic and Iron Ages, along with increased signs of infection, iron deficiency anemia, and developmental delays (Rathburn 1984). Such changes were not immediately apparent when agriculture first began in the Levant region of the Middle East, but skeletal evidence reveals marked declines in nutrition, growth, and development with the later intensification of farming and animal husbandry (Smith 1984). Population pressure clearly preceded the intensification of agriculture in the Eastern Mediterranean, which was then followed by soil depletion, increased protein, iron, and zinc deficiencies, and increased parasitic infections from 1500 BCE until the Classical Period (Angel 1984). Similarly, there is clear evidence for population pressure preceding intensification in South Asia. Evidence for similar sequences of population pressure, agricultural intensification, and subsequent health declines has been found in excavated ancient populations located in present day China, Vietnam, Panama, Peru, and in the eastern and mid-western United States (Price and Gebauer 1995; Cohen and Armelagos 1984).

Among the known transitional societies, two examples stand out which provide the most comprehensive bioarchaeological evidence. The first example is a population of Sudanese Nubians uncovered in thirty-three excavations over a period of seventy years (Martin et al. 1984). These excavations span five major time periods beginning with late Mesolithic foragers in 11 500 BCE and ending with highly agrarian Christians in 1350 CE. Here, there is an eighteenfold increase in dental caries and the first significant evidence of iron deficiency anemia during the early stages of agriculture in the Mesolithic and Neolithic periods (11 500–3400 BCE). These trends continue from 3400 BCE to 350 BCE, along with an overall decrease in stature, with increasing dependence on agriculture and export crops. From this point forward, enamel hypoplasias provide significant evidence of developmental delays in childhood. During the same period, young adult women display premature osteoporosis: a likely sign that lactating women were compensating for nutritional deficiencies by shunting calcium from their bones to their breast milk. It is notable, however, that these Nubian populations show few osteological signs of bacterial infections, despite all other indications of physiological susceptibility. But these latter findings are explained by a unique cultural phenomenon: the ingestion of significant quantities of tetracycline compounds that were most likely present in bread or beer (Bassett et al. 1980). We will examine this phenomenon again when we turn to the history and prehistory of antibiotic use in Chapter 6.

The second comprehensive example is found in a series of excavations at the Dickson Mounds burial complex of southern Illinois, located in the mid-western United States. Here, the archaeological record reveals a small society that had experienced a relatively rapid transformation to intensive maize agriculture. During the Late Woodland Period (950–1100 CE) the site provided a seasonal campsite for 75–100 nomadic foragers. Over the next century, these people became increasingly influenced by their Middle Mississippian neighbors, a large group of over 30 000 sedentary agriculturalists living 180 kilometers to the south (Fowler 1997). By the following century, known as the Middle Mississippian Period (1200–1300 CE), these former woodland foragers had settled into 234 hamlet structures with support camps and work structures for 600–1200 people (Harn 1978). This same period saw the intensification of maize agriculture as a primary means of subsistence, the intensification of trade with neighboring communities, and a marked increase in population size and density.

As with the previous examples, the Dickson Mounds population experienced significant health declines during their transition from nomadic foraging to sedentary agriculture. Yet the evidence from this example is distinctive in at least two ways. First, we can determine that the Dickson Mounds transition occurred within a somewhat genetically isolated population. Where measured, the other examples revealed varying degrees of in-migration from genetically unrelated populations during their transitions. Such migrations open the possibility, however slim, that all these genetic changes were disadvantageous insofar as they increased people's susceptibility to disease. But in the case of Dickson Mounds, comparisons of inherited dental traits confirms that these changes were not due to the in-migration of new groups (Cohen 2009). The same genetic population, clearly distinguishable from neighboring groups, had made the transition from seasonal nomadism to a more sedentary lifestyle over a period of 250 years.

Second, we are able to employ nearly all known health measurements to the Dickson Mounds populations throughout the transition period. While most of the previous examples provide different subsets of health data at different time periods, Dickson Mounds yields a comprehensive set of measurements across a continuum of time and changes in lifestyle. The result is a very thorough record of health changes, such as a fourfold increase in iron deficiency anemia accompanying an overall decrease in stature and cortical bone thickness. Enamel hypoplasias reveal developmental interruptions in childhood, and we see overall declines in life expectancy for every age interval. There are also significant increases in traumatic injuries and degenerative spinal problems. Most significantly, the Dickson Mounds transition accompanied more than a threefold increase in the periosteal signs of bacterial infections.

These results bear further analysis. Much of the evidence for iron deficiency anemia at Dickson Mounds can be found in young children, a condition associated with a two to six month decrease in life expectancy during the first ten years of life. The impact of periosteal reactions on life expectancy is even more severe: children born with these signs of infection have a 50 per cent decrease in life expectancy in comparison with other children in the same populations. Furthermore, the evidence for anemia and bacterial infections not only track together at Dickson Mounds, but in many instances these diseases are present in the same individuals. In these cases, both diseases are much more severe, a finding consistent with the well-known association between nutritional deficiencies and immune deficiencies—a syndemic so often found in the world's impoverished societies today.

Even for those who survived these childhood diseases, the risk of further infection would have been greatly increased by permanent impairments in immune system development. Much of this development, such as the maturation of the thymus and lymph system, occurs in the first four years of life. These are the same years in which we see signs of growth impairment in long bones and vertebral canals, the latter being a particular sign of delays during a critical period of immune system development. We also see earlier signs of enamel hypoplasias, which in turn indicate earlier ages of weaning—a major risk factor for childhood infections, and one that correlates with signs of calcium deficiency in women of childbearing ages. Given these data, there is little wonder that a fifteen-year-old post-agricultural Mississippian could expect to live eighteen fewer years than his or her foraging ancestor of the same age (Cohen 1977). These patterns are consistent with observations of contemporary living populations, in which low birth weight and early childhood hardships result in greater disease susceptibility throughout adulthood (Kuzawa and Quinn 2009; Barker 2004). For these societies, agriculture came at a significant cost.

2.3 Selecting for Infectious Diseases

The weight and extent of the bioarchaeological evidence leaves little doubt that the intensification of agriculture brought health changes to ancient human populations. It should be noted, however, that despite significant differences between pre- and post-transition societies, the direction of these changes is not immediately obvious from simple comparisons of skeletal pathologies. An alternative interpretation of this evidence, known as the Osteological Paradox, states that the higher frequency of pathologies in agricultural populations may actually reflect improvements in their overall health (Wood et al. 1992). The reasoning follows that being healthier, ancient agricultural societies were better able to survive diseases and other hardships than their foraging predecessors, thereby accumulating more pathologies over longer average lifespans. These pathologies could then be a sign of greater toughness in the face of hardship, rather than a sign of greater hardship itself.

The evidence for toughness may be no better than the evidence for sickness, but the prospect of an Osteological Paradox prompts us to consider how opposite conclusions could be drawn from the same data. Faced with this challenge, we can rule out the paradox only when we consider the archaeological evidence in the context of people's life histories. This is where the age data for these populations are particularly helpful. First, in all instances where we can reasonably determine the general ages of skeletons, we see that more people die earlier with agricultural as opposed to foraging lifestyles—a strong indication of declining health with sedentism and agriculture. Second, we know that peak frequencies of pathology in early childhood are commonly associated with populations facing higher rates of infection and other health problems, and we know they are commonly associated with earlier ages of death (Goodman and Armelagos 1988). We can therefore safely conclude that the higher frequencies of pathology in agricultural populations is indeed associated with health declines rather than health improvements.

Yet even when they confirm health problems, these data are circumstantial insofar as they merely confirm an association between the intensification of agriculture and an increasing burden of disease; they do not confirm that agriculture is the actual cause of these diseases. To make a better case for causality, we must also examine direct evidence for those broader lifestyle changes that are known to affect human health and disease, especially with regards to the evolution of potential human pathogens. For this, we revisit the same themes of subsistence, settlement, and social organization that we addressed for nomadic foragers in the previous chapter.

With respect to dietary subsistence, ancient pollen and spore samples provide direct evidence of decreasing nutritional diversity with the intensification of agriculture. We find this in South Asia, where the intensification of agriculture stabilized the seasonal availability of food, but did so with the restriction of edible plant resources (Kennedy 1984). Similarly, the expansion of agriculture in the Mediterranean was accompanied by the overuse of soil through monocropping (Angel 1984). As they began settling into permanent residences, the Mississippians of Dickson Mounds became increasingly dependent on a single staple crop, maize, for their caloric intake (Martin et al. 1984). Although maize is a great source of nutritional energy, it is deficient in zinc and the amino acid lysine, both of which are essential for healthy immune function. These crop data constitute an important missing link in the chain of causality between subsistence practices and susceptibility to infectious diseases.

Regarding settlement patterns, we not only see the expansion of populations with agriculture, but more importantly, the concentration of populations in permanent settlement clusters. Indeed, the correlation of agriculture with increasing population size and density has led some anthropologists to argue that sedentism, more than agriculture per se, was the primary trigger for the first emergence of acute human infections (Cohen and Armelagos 1984). We know that this settlement theory is supported by studies that we examined in the previous chapter. But it is difficult to weigh settlement above other factors without first determining its precise location in the sequence of causality. For instance, we have many archaeological finds in which the size and density of human populations preceded the further intensification of agriculture. But we do not know if these kinds of population pressure might, in turn, be the result of earlier changes of subsistence. Subsistence and settlement changes were clearly linked to one another, but they are chickens and eggs; it is impossible to determine which came first.

Less obvious is the impact of agriculture on the settlement of nonhuman animals. Whether for meat or for labor, the domestication of animals increased the size and densities of animal populations, just as it did for their human handlers. It also brought them into close proximity with one another, and it did so for longer periods of time than when we hunted our meat in the wild. Combining these factors created a "perfect storm" for the spread of zoonotic diseases from animal to human hosts. Thus, it is with little surprise that we find most major human infections have their evolutionary origins as zoonotic diseases (Weiss 2001).

Here, we find evidence tracing the origins of smallpox and tuberculosis to domesticated ruminants. Smallpox is related to cowpox, one variant of which is the *vaccinia* strain that has long been used to inoculate the human race against the more virulent disease. The measles virus originated with the rinderpest virus in cattle, which most likely made the leap to human populations in the 11–12th Centuries (Furuse et al. 2010). Phylogenetic studies of all influenzas, human and otherwise, show that all are essentially avian influenzas insofar as they all thrive in the guts of waterfowl that have been variously domesticated by a number of human societies (Alexander 2000). All of these animal origins make sense in the light of the opportunities provided by sedentism and the domestication of livestock. In later chapters, we will see how new viruses can enter the human population by the exchange of blood and body fluids through the hunting and butchering of wild animals. However, the added risk of domestication is that it necessitates the same kinds of exchange opportunities, but does so over much longer and sustained periods of time. By placing humans and animals in close proximity to themselves, as well as to one another, agriculture creates repeated opportunities for the transmission of pathogens.

Lastly, we can consider the evidence for health-related changes in social organizations associated with agriculture. In the previous examples, we have seen evidence that women suffered disproportionately with the intensification of agriculture. These differences were even more striking with political centralization. In the case of the Sudanese Nubian populations, life expectancies were inversely correlated with the degree of centralization, and notably, with the effects more pronounced among women and other subgroups living on the periphery of major political centers (Van Gerven et al. 1990). Ironically, these health declines were lowest among these groups during the same periods that the Nubian kingdoms of Meroë (ca. 800 BCE–350 CE) and Makuria (ca. 500–700 CE) were at their heights of wealth and power. Such associations are best explained by these kingdoms exerting greater control over their populations to extract additional labor and resources from peripheral subgroups— a common theme in human history and the global inequalities of the present day. Interestingly, we see signs of improved health in these same subgroups during the decline and collapse of these kingdoms.

Just as we can see health differences between different groups of ancient skeletons, so too can we see social and economic differences according to the manner in which they are buried. It is reasonable to infer that people buried with valuable objects in larger and more elaborate graves are of a higher status than those with few or no objects buried in small and simple graves. Such differences are most apparent when comparing royalty with their subjects, but the same logic can be applied to other strata of hierarchical societies. Such differences become increasingly apparent with the intensification of agriculture in the Dickson Mounds populations of Illinois (Buikstra 1984). When these data are correlated with skeletal data, we see that socio-economic status is positively associated with better nutrition and growth, just as it is inversely associated with signs of infectious disease. Moreover, these differences in health and disease are most pronounced when comparing groups of people who were buried with at least some decorative artifacts with those who were buried with nothing at all.

We find the same associations in the skeletons and graves of historical populations throughout the world (Armelagos et al. 2005; Paynter and McGuire 1991). Indeed, it is a story as old as human hierarchy, and one that continues to be told in the present day: people with greater resources tend to be relatively healthier than people with lesser resources. Societies having greater resource differences will also tend to have greater health differences, and so on. But it is important to note that although these differences can be traced to prehistoric antiquity, they not as old as humanity itself. Rather, they are the more recent results of the Agricultural Revolution. Combined with declining nutritional quality, increasing population density, and proximity to nonhuman animals, these social changes brought the first major rises of acute infectious diseases in the human species.

2.4 Europe and the People without Smallpox

From the Neolithic Revolution to the Industrial Revolution, the First Transition spread across the world like a plague of plagues. In its wake came the first truly emerging infections as the primary cause of death in sedentary societies, with the greatest impact on the very young and the very poor, and the greatest concentrations in the urban centers of expanding empires. It was not long before these emerging infections became endemic infections, persistent problems that came to be seen as inevitable fixtures of human life. Indeed, it would have been difficult to remember things any other way, since only sedentary societies would have had the means to store written records over long periods of time. Even our early disease histories came from people already well accustomed to acute infections: Heroditus' on dysentery among the Persian Army, Procopius on the Justinian Plague, Bonaiuti on the Black Death (Bray 1996). While these authors appreciated the dramatic scope of these pandemics, they did so from a baseline of day-to-day infections that would most likely have led to their own demise. Under these conditions, the popular truism that "history is written by the victors"[6] acquires a special meaning. Until the Industrial Revolution, the history of disease was written by societies who themselves bore the greatest burden of acute infections. Disease was written by the infected.

Written history notwithstanding, we know from the archaeological record that the Agricultural Revolution arose independently in different geographic centers and historical periods. We also know that it was adopted at different rates and different degrees by surrounding communities as it spread out from these centers. It therefore follows that these communities would have had different experiences of the First Epidemiological Transition, with disease rates determined by particular sociocultural circumstances. Societies that were more socially stratified, those that were more densely settled, and those that depended on a more restricted set of domesticated foods, would have had higher rates of infectious diseases than those that were less stratified, more widely settled, and better nourished.

This was the case for disease differences between Old and New World populations prior to the European invasion of the Americas. In the years following Columbus' first landing at Hispanola in 1492, Europeans systematically massacred, enslaved, and forcibly displaced native populations across the Americas (Watts 1997). At the same time, they introduced Old World diseases such as smallpox, typhoid, and measles—infections that rapidly spread alongside organized violence throughout the New World, leading to the death of more than 50 million Native Americans—the majority of human life on two continents (Crosby 2003; Dobyns 1993; Ramenofsky 1987).

Viewed from the perspective of epidemiological transitions, the European invasion of the Americas represents a sudden and violent collision of pre- and post-transition societies on a global scale. Some explanations focus on the biological aspects of this collision, proposing "virgin soil" arguments in which Native Americans were immunologically under-equipped to deal with European infections (Crosby 1976). Other explanations focus on the ways that violence produced selective conditions for infectious diseases (Watts 1997). Of course, neither of these explanations need diminish the other in any way. Indeed, we would argue that the Native American genocide was a *syndemic* of violence and infection: a perfect storm produced by the biosocial interactions between these factors that produced far greater mortality than either could alone.

---

[6] This statement is often attributed to Winston Churchill, although there is no documentation to confirm it.

To better appreciate these dynamics, we must first consider the ancient ancestors of Native American populations: the so-called "Paleo Indians" who first crossed the Siberian land bridge from northern Asia toward the end of the last Ice Age and prior to the first Agricultural Revolution. Archaeologists debate the timing of the very first migrations, which may have occurred as early as 40 000 years ago (Goebel et al. 2008). But genetic studies of contemporary AmerIndian populations indicate that their biological ancestors stemmed from a few, relatively small Siberian populations who most likely entered the New World between 13 000 and 17 000 years ago, a period encompassing the Clovis complex, the earliest-known tools in the Americas (Waters and Stafford 2007; Schurr 2004). There may have been earlier waves of migration, but these were the people who ultimately populated the Americas before Columbus' arrival.

At the time of these migrations, the chain of Aleutian Islands between Siberia and Alaska were the high ground of a continuous land bridge known as Beringia. This ancient land bridge was a relatively ice-free zone that presented good hunting and living opportunities for nomadic foraging groups. Following such opportunities, these groups eventually radiated throughout the American continents.

The PaleoIndian migrations have at least two important implications for disease susceptibility among historical Native American populations. The first is that relatively small numbers of initial migrants produced a genetic bottleneck such that their future descendants would share many traits in common. The second implication is that the living conditions of these first migrants were very much like the hunting and gathering groups we described in the previous chapter. Their diets consisted of lean game meat and very fibrous plant materials—a situation that has led some researchers to hypothesize a "thrifty-gene" coding for sensitive insulin receptors that could more easily process carbohydrates under conditions of limited availability (Neel 1982). That same sensitivity could result in a higher risk for adult onset diabetes if the same biological populations suddenly found themselves surrounded by excess carbohydrates in the form of cheap and fast food. This Thrifty-Gene hypothesis has been used to explain unusually high rates of diabetes in many acculturated Native American populations (Hales and Barker 2001).[7]

As we saw in Chapter 1, it is very difficult for acute infectious diseases to maintain themselves in small, geographically scattered populations. It is therefore unlikely that PaleoIndian migrants faced many such diseases. Even in later years, when many groups settled down and began farming, the trade and social networks between groups was nowhere near as extensive in the Americas as in the Eurasian continents. Globalization was already well underway in the Old World by the 5th century CE, with trade routes linking Mongolia with Western Europe and North Africa (McNeill 1976). In comparison, even the great nation states of the Inca, the Maya, and the Aztec did not typically extend their reach by more than a thousand miles. While there were certainly post-First Transition societies in the Americas, many more pre-transition societies had not been exposed to the varieties of acute infections found in densely settled populations. So while the PaleoIndians may have once shared the same disease ecology with their European counterparts tens of thousands of years ago, this was no longer the case at the time of their descendants' tragic reunion.

---

[7] Hales and Barker specifically argue for a thrifty phenotype resulting from fetal stress. However, this article also provides a good review of the topic more broadly.

This brings us to the virgin soil arguments for differences in disease susceptibility between Old World and New World populations. To date, there is no genetic evidence that contemporary Native Americans have inherited any unusual susceptibility to infections of European origin (Jones 2003). That said, it appears that Native Americans have less diversity in certain genetic regions that code for key immune molecules known as the Major Histocompatibility Complex (MHC) or Human Leukocyte Antigen (HLA) system. A comparative sample of different geographic populations finds that Native Americans have fewer than half the variant forms (known as alleles) for these genetic regions than other Old World populations (Black 1992).

Based on these data, it follows that a pathogen, having adapted to a particular MHC allele within a host, would be more likely adapt to another host having the same MHC allele than it would to a host having a different MHC allele. Thus, in a Native American population with less MHC diversity, a pathogen would be more likely to encounter the same MHC alleles and therefore show higher transmission and virulence. With this in mind, it is certainly possible that greater MHC diversity in Old World human populations may reflect a micro-evolutionary adaption to disease conditions following the First Transition that would not be shared by pre-transition New World populations. However, it should also be noted that, while MHC variability may have been a contributing factor to differential mortality, it is by no means sufficient to explain more than 50 million Native American deaths.

A more compelling version of the virgin soil argument focuses more on developmental rather than genetic differences. The human immune system develops much of its defenses through exposure to pathogens. Each new exposure results in the production of memory cells that allow the immune system to mount a more rapid and robust response should the host encounter the same pathogen, or similar pathogens, in the future. In many cases, the host need only have a mild or sub-clinical (i.e. symptom free) infection to acquire immunity to more virulent forms of the pathogen. This same principle of acquired immunity governs the efficacy of live vaccines. It could also govern the differential immunity of pre- and post-transition populations.

Now consider the disease conditions of late 15th-century Europe, a time when children often died from infections before reaching adulthood. Those that survived would have acquired defenses to numerous pathogens, such that they would be little affected even when sharing close quarters with asymptomatic carriers on a long sea voyage. Under these conditions, one would expect that these same, otherwise attenuated infections could have a disastrous effect on a previously unexposed population. There are even European precedents for this kind of virgin soil epidemic. When smallpox struck the Scottish island of Foula in 1720, it killed almost 95 per cent of its inhabitants, an isolated population in which no one had been previously exposed to the disease (Watts 1997). Similar epidemics killed 90 per cent of the indigenous Mesoamerican and Andean populations (Dobyns 1993).

Despite these compelling examples, there are at least two problems with explanations that rely solely on acquired immunity. The first is that virgin soil epidemics do not usually kill the majority of their host populations. The Black Death, often thought to be the quintessential virgin soil epidemic, probably resulted in no more than 30 per cent mortality (Watts 1997). Similar rates have been found in more recent epidemics among unexposed Native American groups. The Great Alaskan Sickness of 1900, which was probably a combination of measles and influenza, killed about 25 per cent of the western native population (Wolfe 1982). And a 1952 measles epidemic in isolated Amazonian populations of Brazil resulted in about 36 per cent mortality (Crosby 1976). Of course, these are devastating statistics; it is difficult to fathom the human toll of losing a third of one's family, friends, and community. Yet even so, these losses do not approach those of the Native Americans in the period between the 15th and 17th centuries.

It may be that the combined effects of multiple European diseases were overwhelming to the point that they nearly extinguished indigenous life in the New World. But this rejoinder still leaves a second and far more intractable problem: most Native American groups never regained their original numbers. Even three to four generations after the end of these epidemics, when most groups would have acquired at least as much immunity to the European infections as the Europeans themselves, the Native American populations remained a fraction of their pre-contact sizes. No lack of immunity, inherited or acquired, could account for this phenomenon.

This leaves us to consider the biological impact of violence, subjugation, and forced displacement. In addition to causing direct casualties, these forced actions produce the most fertile conditions for infectious diseases: starvation, stress, poor sanitation, social disruption, and crowding. We see this time and again with refugee populations of the present day, which often serve as the most sensitive reservoirs for virulent and drug-resistant infections. It is therefore unsurprising that the combination of violence and novel infection would have such devastating effects on human populations, and that the persistence of the former would impede the demographic recovery of these same populations.

William McNeill coined the term "macroparasitism" to describe stiuations when one group acquires food and energy at the expense of the other (McNeill 1976). The European invasion of the Americas was a clear case of macroparasitism that also brought new microparasites to pre-transition societies. The Native American genocide can thus be seen as a syndemic of two organismic categories: one microbial, the other human.

Disease historians commonly refer to these events as the "Columbian exchange," for although the Transatlantic interactions were grossly unequal, they nevertheless resulted in the transmission of new infections in both directions. Europe brought dozens of pathogenic microbes across the Atlantic, but they also returned with a few New World pathogens. The most notorious of these was syphilis. The first identifiable European outbreak occurred in 1495, shortly after Columbus' return. After laying siege to Naples, the French and mercenary armies of Charles VII returned to their homes with the telltale chancre sores on their genitalia, later followed by diffuse rashes on their hands and feet (Harper et al. 2011). The infection quickly spread throughout Europe, and the following years revealed worst signs of the disease: inflammatory tumors, bone degeneration, paralysis, blindness, insanity, and death— the novelty and severity of which is indicative of a virgin soil epidemic. Named for the unfortunate shepherd and protagonist of Fracastoro's 16th-century poem, and alternatively referred to as the French, Spanish, and Neopolitan disease, Syphilis had become the AIDS of Renaissance Europe (Quetel et al. 1990).

Despite its sudden appearance in European history, there has been a great deal of debate regarding the geographic origin and antiquity of syphilis (Armelagos and Baker 1988; Harper et al. 2011). Adding to this controversy, the spirochete bacterium responsible for syphilis, *Treponema pallidum pallidum*, is one of four nearly indistinguishable subspecies. The other three are responsible for non-venereal infections that are often contracted in childhood through oral or skin-to-skin contact. *T. pallidum pertinue* produces yaws, an infection of the skin, bones, and joints found in moist tropical climates. *T. pallidum endemicum* produces similar signs in a disease known as bejel, which is found in hot and arid environments. The fourth and most unique among the treponemal infections, *T. pallidum carateum*, produces the relative mild skin effects of pinta, which is only found in Central and South America.

Based on these microbial ambiguities, some researchers have argued for a pre-Columbian hypothesis whereby treponemal infections had long existed in the Old World, buried among similar skin diseases that often bore the ancient moniker of "leprosy" (Cockburn 1967). In accordance with this hypothesis, these could have been relatively mild infections until economic changes brought increased population densities, thereby selecting for the evolution of an acute, virulent, hardier (and therefore venereal) form of the disease. It should be noted, however, that this evolutionary scenario could also apply to a newly imported organism, as per the Columbian hypothesis, or a combination of organisms on multiple Old World continents, with Paleolithic origins that later followed human migrations to the New World much like the other souvenir parasites described in the previous chapter (Kliks 1990).

However interesting these alternative arguments, the paleopathological and genetic evidence strongly supports a New World origin for syphilis. The majority of skeletal lesions in late-stage treponemal infections display a "worm-eaten" appearance, known as caries sicca, in the outer table of the cranial vault. There is also symmetrical destruction of the bone surrounding the nasal area, and significant periosteal reaction in the tibia that often involves a thickening and deformation of the bone itself (Armelagos and Baker 1988). While it is impossible to diagnose whether these pathologies are specifically due to syphilis, bejel, or yaws, they can nevertheless be distinguished from pathologies found in severe forms of leprosy or bone tuberculosis. To-date, there is no unequivocal skeletal evidence of treponemal infections in Europe before the 15th century. There is, however, ample skeletal evidence in prehistorical New World populations.

Even more convincing, evidence comes from a phylogenetic study that compares the relatedness of twenty-six treponemal strains from multiple geographic locations (Harper et al. 2008). This analysis reveals that all the syphilis strains have the most recent evolutionary origins. Furthermore, these syphilis strains were more closely related to the yaws strains from South America than to all the other non-venereal strains. Old World yaws strains revealed the oldest evolutionary origins. From these data, it appears that non-venereal treponemal infections arose first in the Old World and eventually spread to the New World, but that syphilis arose from the latter New World strains. Thus, it could be said that Columbus and colleagues brought new pathogens to unexposed populations on both sides of the Atlantic. But the exchange was far from even.

Part Two

The Second Transition

3

Why Germ Theory Didn't Matter

There is an Hour when I must die,
Nor do I know how soon 'twill come;
A thousand Children young as I
Are call'd by Death to hear their Doom.

Divine Songs. *Isaac Watts (1715)*

No parent should ever have to bury a child. Yet until the 20th century, this was an all too-common experience for parents in settled societies around the world. It was even common for English parents during the height of the British Empire, a time when child elegies were a popular form of verse. This genre culminated in the late Victorian era with "comfort books" designed to help grieving mothers come to terms with the loss of their children (Jalland 1996). Many of these books tried to ease the pain with platitudes about heroism, early salvation, and playmates in heaven. Others went on to wrestle with the tragedy and injustice of premature death. Emily Dickinson invoked both these narratives when she envisioned a graveyard as a ghostly playground where "[t]here was a figure plump for every little knoll," while also remarking how "feet so precious charged should reach so small a goal" (Dickinson 1896: I, 146). Indeed, a large proportion of graveyards in this era were populated with the little knolls of foreshortened lives.

Such tragedies were reflected in the statistics of the time. In the years just prior to 1840, three out of ten English children died before they reached the age of fifteen (Wrigley et al. 1997). Between 1800 and 1840, only 44 per cent of London children survived to twenty-five years of age. With an average of five children per family, an English mother was likely to lose at least one son or daughter before he or she reached adulthood. Nor was England an exception in this regard; indeed, child mortality was significantly worse in many other countries, but until the late 19th century, no other country measured its tragedies so rigorously. England systematically recorded its fertility and mortality rates in relation to life tables, and created standardized criteria for determining causes of death, all of which allowed the country to amass the world's most reliable health statistics from 1841–1911. These statistics revealed that infectious diseases were the overwhelming causes of death and that most of these deaths occurred in childhood (Eyler 1979).

Not long after the English began collecting health statistics, their mortality figures began showing overall declines. These declines were slow at first, with a gradual leveling of "crisis"

An Unnatural History of Emerging Infections. First Edition. Ron Barrett and George J. Armelagos
© Ron Barrett and George J. Armelagos 2013. Published 2013 by Oxford University Press.

peaks that had reflected earlier, periodic epidemics. Then the mortality baselines themselves began trending downward until they fell precipitously in the early 20th century. Similar trends could be seen in other affluent nations during the same time periods. These declines were so dramatic that they drove an exponential rise in the total human population of the world—this, despite overall fertility declines. During the same period, chronic degenerative diseases replaced infectious diseases as the primary causes of death. These health and demographic changes constitute the "Classic Model" of Abdel Omran's Transition Theory (Omran 1971). We call it the Second Epidemiological Transition.

The mortality declines of the Second Transition were the first of their magnitude since the Neolithic. Perhaps more surprising, the largest portion of these declines occurred before the widespread acceptance of Germ Theory and well before the discovery of antibiotics and most vaccines. Although Germ Theory eventually led to many important medical discoveries, most of these arose well after the major ebb of disease-causing pathogens from affluent societies. In Chapter 2, we examined the tragic consequences of the First Epidemiological Transition, which strongly implicated the human determinants of under-nutrition, the crowding of people and animals, as well as social inequalities and concomitant violence. This chapter examines the positive side of the same coin when these human determinants reverse themselves to some degree. Such reversals hold important lessons about the best ways to approach new, virulent, and drug-resistant infections today, provided we also improve the distribution and use of newer medical technologies.

3.1 Germ Theory versus the Sanitary Reform Movement

The Germ Theory of disease causation is based on ancient ideas that were not adopted by the Western biomedical establishment until the last decades of the 19th century. Even then, most biomedical physicians converted only gradually and grudgingly after decades of contentious debates. Germ Theory made sporadic appearances in post-classical Western societies. Writing in the 1st century BCE, Marcus Torentius Varro warned that "in swampy places minute creatures live that cannot be discerned with the eye and they enter the body through the mouth and nostrils and cause serious disease" (Varro 1783/1934: L.1,12,2). Girolamo Fracastoro, the same Renaissance scholar who coined the term "syphilis," proposed a similar idea about contagion in the 16th century (Fracastoro 1530). Fracastoro suggested that diseases are caused by invisible "semenaria," the translation of which was probably the first use of "germ" in this context. But it was not until late in the next century that Anton van Leeuwenhoek developed a microscope of sufficient resolution to observe unicellular organisms for the first time (Dobell 1932). Even then, the medical establishment viewed his observations with a great deal of skepticism.

Prior to the adoption of Germ Theory, most biomedical physicians believed that fever diseases were caused by miasma—poisonous gasses emitted by the putrefaction of organic matter such as feces or rotting plants and animals. Even by the middle of the 19th century, with the Industrial Revolution well underway in Europe and North America, there were good reasons for the Western medical establishment's leaning more toward miasmic contamination than germ contagion when dealing with the most lethal infections of the day. To begin with, the evidence was still ambiguous. Even with improved microscopes, it was difficult to clearly visualize these supposed microorganisms, and all the more daunting to clearly identify particular varieties and then link them to particular diseases. Such links have sometimes been difficult to prove with today's technology; the technical challenges were far greater in the 1850s and 1860s.

Germ Theory was also strongly associated with the late medieval practice of quarantine, a prospect that was not well-received in post-Enlightenment times. Derived from the Venetian *quaranta giorni* (forty days), the quarantine applied the Old Testament practice of forced isolation, not only to persons in transit, but also to entire communities and anyone under suspicion during the Black Death (Perri 2008). By the beginning of the 15th century, quarantines had become widely adopted by European nations, becoming emblems of church and state bureaucracy. Such emblems clashed with the economic and ideological transformations of Renaissance Europe, and even more with its free-market industries several centuries later. Certainly, no commercial port or shipping company had an interest in adopting regular quarantines that would impede the flow of goods and capital.

Quarantines also presented an empirical problem for Germ Theory when applied to infectious diseases that are not directly transmitted by human-to-human contact. Speaking against "contagionism" in 1834, J. A. Rouchoux cited the failure of quarantines to contain the yellow fever and typhus epidemics during the Napoleonic Wars (Rouchoux 1834). Both were vector-borne diseases that relied on insects to transmit their respective pathogens between humans: typhus being transmitted by lice, and yellow fever by the mosquito *Aedes egypticus*. No quarantine could contain such tiny creatures, and even the contagionists of the time did not suspect the role of insects in the transmission of pathogens across human boundaries.

The same could be said for water and food-borne diseases such as typhoid and cholera, which could pass freely along plumbing and trade networks, affecting thousands without anyone ever coming into direct contact with other infected people. That said, John Snow famously demonstrated the water-borne transmission of cholera with medical geography and health statistics (Johnson 2006; Snow 1855) (see Figure 3.1). Working in partnership with William Farr in the General Register Office, Snow analyzed London mortality data for two cholera epidemics, the latter of which spared a large set of previously affected neighborhoods when, during the years between the epidemics, the company supplying their drinking water had shifted its intake pipes further upstream along the Thames River.[1] Yet although this struck a blow to the airborne nature of miasma, in many cases it merely changed peoples' views about the medium of transmission rather than the deadly message itself. It did not necessarily follow that cholera was caused by living organisms.

[1] John Snow is famously credited for identifying the source of a neighborhood cholera outbreak at the Broad Street water pump in London, and then having the handle of the pump removed so no water could be drawn, and thus ingested, from that particular well. It should be noted, however, that the epidemic was already waning by the time of its removal. Furthermore, the Broad Street study, while poignant, was part of a much larger statistical comparison of two epidemics throughout the greater London area. This comparison, which Snow dubbed "The Grand Experiment," provided convincing evidence that the disease was transmitted by water (Johnson 2006).

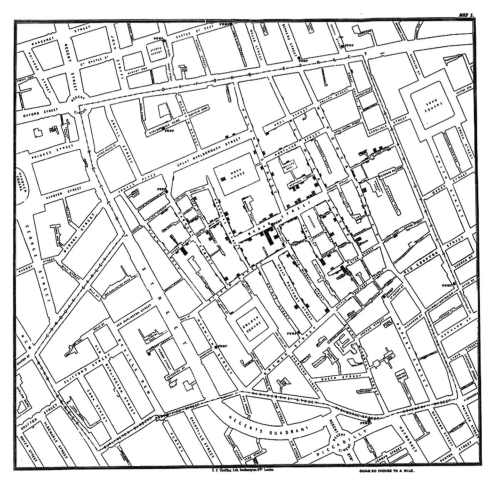

Figure 3.1. John Snow's original map depicting a geographic cluster of cholera cases in the Broad Street area of London during the 1854 epidemic. This was part of a much larger statistical comparison of two cholera epidemics that demonstrated the water-borne contagion of the disease. Snow, John 1855. *On the Mode of Communication of Cholera.* 2nd Ed. London: Churchill.

Quarantines and vectors aside, the strongest case against Germ Theory was based on the success of the sanitarians, who were usually strong believers of miasma. Despite their mistaken etiology, the sanitarians promoted a set of public health interventions that were highly effective at preventing many infectious diseases. Believing dirt and decay to be the origin of the deadly gases, their major agenda were aimed at achieving cleaner living conditions. The Sanitary Reform Movement focused on community health through infrastructural improvements in waste disposal, water quality, drainage, and ventilation. The movement also focused on personal cleanliness, not only through improved hygiene, but also by the curtailing of vices (Eyler 1979; Walkowitz 1982).

Sanitarians also made good use of statistics. Florence Nightingale was among the most famous reformers and health statisticians of her day (Nightingale 1859/1992). In addition to her training as a nurse, Nightingale learned quantitative methods under the tutelage of Adolph Quetelet (Diamond 1981; Quetelet 1842). She employed these methods during the Crimean War, when she brought her team of nurses to the Scutari Barracks military hospital in Istanbul (Kopf 1916). Informed by Miasma Theory and applying its sanitary methods, Nightingale's team cleaned up the hospital wards, regularly bathed the patients and changed their linens, created a separate supply chain, and brought in new cooks and menus to ensure better nutrition (McDonald 2001). They also opened the windows for ventilation and ensured that the soldiers received regular mail to boost their morale. Nightingale kept careful records throughout her mission, keeping mortality tables and drawing up "coxcomb" charts that illustrated dramatic reductions in patient death rates (see Figure 3.2). Beginning from a baseline mortality of 43 per cent, the patient death rate dropped to 2 per cent within six months of instituting her reforms. Nightingale's data impressed the War Department, and her reforms were implemented by military units throughout the British Empire. They also gave credence to reforms at home, although not without some political controversy (see Kudzma 2006).

Of course, the germ theorists supported most of the same sanitation principles as the miasmists. After all, the acknowledgement of microbes reinforced the virtues of clean environments for preventing disease transmission. Sir Joseph Lister famously presented one such example. Taking up a recommendation published by Louis Pasteur in the early 1870s, Lister

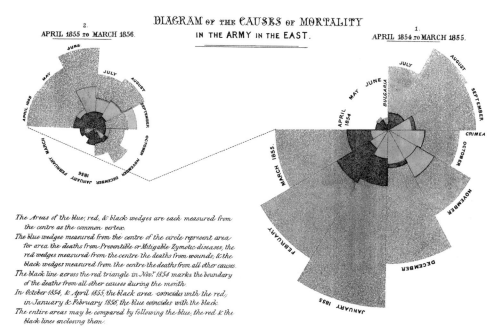

Figure 3.2. Florence Nightingale's coxcomb chart depicting the decline in mortality of Brith soldiers at Scutari hospital before and after her reforms from April 1855 to March 1856. The light-grey portion (blue on the original) represents "preventable deaths" that were likely due to infectious diseases. Nightingale, Florence 1858. *Notes on Matters Affecting the Health, Efficiency, and Hospital Administration of the British Army.* London: Harrison & Sons.

instituted antiseptic measures in his surgical practice that were soon adopted by surgeons around the world (Broughton et al. 2006). Yet outside the operating theater, the miasmists had already made a name for their role in sanitary reform, and they continued to dominate the leadership of major programs and policies aimed at disease prevention. Germ theorists had begun a revolution in medical thinking, but in the realm of medical practice, they could do little more than agree with the existing recommendations of the miasmists.

Undoubtedly, the last decades of the 19th century were exciting times for microbiology. Improved microscopes and staining techniques were revealing microbes that had been previously unobservable, and an emerging guild of microbiologists were systematically demonstrating the associations between these organisms and particular diseases. Louis Pasteur discovered the bacterial origins of fermentation and food spoilage. Robert Koch developed a set of postulates for demonstrating bacterial disease transmission and applied these postulates to identify the bacilli responsible for anthrax, cholera, and tuberculosis (Brock, 1988: 184). Others followed; among them Alexandre Yersin identified the plague bacillus, and Armauer Hansen, the leprosy bacillus (Hansen and Looft 1895; Yersin 1894).

These were important and exciting discoveries, yet with the exception of a few vaccines and surgical asepsis, Germ Theory offered little in the way of new developments for the practice of medicine until well into the 20th century. In the interim, the advice of the sanitarians held sway. Regardless of whether they believed in bacterial or miasmatic causes, most biomedical physicians at the time prescribed nutrition and a clean environment as the primary treatments for infectious diseases. Such prescriptions were well-founded, as they were largely responsible for the decline of infectious diseases from the beginning of the Second Epidemiological Transition to the end of the Second World War.

3.2 The McKeown Thesis

The Second Epidemiological Transition made its appearance with an unprecedented rise in human populations around the middle of the 17th century (Omran 1971). Prior to this, settled agricultural societies were characterized as having both high fertility rates and high mortality rates, the latter fluctuating with periodic epidemics. People had more children, but these children were born with life expectancies of only 20–40 years, with some years being better or worse than others depending on the occurence of larger than usual infectious disease outbreaks. This long-standing pattern resulted in sporadic cycles of increasing and decreasing populations. Yet on the whole, the cycles pointed gradually upward, with incremental rises in total population over long periods of time. In this manner, the total human population grew slowly, if sporadically, from an estimated 10 million at the time of the Neolithic to about 800 million over the next nine-and-a-half millennia (McKeown 1965).

This was a significant increase, but it was not nearly as dramatic as the exponential rise of human populations over the next three centuries (see Figure 3.3). By 1830, the total human population had reached 1 billion people. It doubled to 2 billion in the next one hundred years, doubled again to 4 billion in the next forty-five years, and then increased to 7 billion in less than forty years to the time of this publication (Livi-Bacci 2012). Even more interesting,

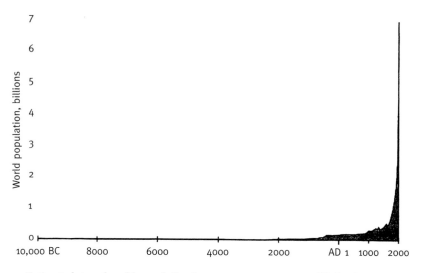

Figure 3.3. Estimated size of world population from 10 000 BCE to 2011 CE. We begin to see exponential population growth in the 18th century. U.S. Census Bureau.

these expansions occurred despite relatively flat, and even downward trends in fertility. Dramatic or not, any population increase can only be caused by one of two factors, or a combination thereof: a) the rate of people added to the population (i.e., fertility); and, b) the rate of people subtracted from the population (i.e., mortality). With fertility rates unchanged or declining, the only remaining explanation is that even greater mortality declines were responsible for the rapid expansion of the human population.

Such was the case among many relatively affluent nations of Europe and North America. We can observe these demographic trends earliest in Scandinavian countries such as Sweden, which began collecting reliable national census data in the middle of the 18th century (McKeown 1976). The Swedish population increased nearly fivefold from 1.76 million in 1749 to 7.4 million in 1950. Swedish birth rates continued to fluctuate around 18th century levels and then fell significantly in the last quartile of the 19th century. From this, we can infer that changing mortality rather than fertility contributed to the population increase.

England and Wales saw an eightfold expansion of their populations from 1700–1950, despite similar fertility declines during the same period (McKeown 1988). It should be noted, however, that the English population data for the 18th century is based on family reconstructions of parish records rather than census data (Eyler 1979). Parishes record baptisms rather than births, and burials rather than deaths. They may miss people who migrate between parishes, and of course, they do not count churchless dissenters. As such, the earlier data on the English and Welsh is not as reliable as that of the Swedes, but that said, the English provided excellent census data after 1841, when population dynamics of the Second Transition were plainly apparent. From this time on, England and Wales provided detailed mortality data based on life tables, which measure the ratio of deaths to the total life years rather than to the total population figure. From these calculations, we see a mortality decline from 25.8 in 1811 to 18.3

in 1871 (McKeown et al. 1972). More importantly, England and Wales provides us with excellent data on mortality by age and by cause after 1838. These data present clear evidence that the mortality decline was chiefly due to falling rates of infection-related deaths, most having occurred in childhood. These populations expanded because more people were either surviving deadly childhood infections or avoiding them altogether.

Based on closer examination of these data, Thomas McKeown, a physician and medical historian, concludes that new medical technologies made little contribution to the decline of infectious diseases in England and Wales in the 19th and early 20th centuries (1976) Convincingly, McKeown illustrates his point with line graphs of changing mortality rates for specific infections, and their temporal relationships to the development of effective biomedical therapies and cures. Tuberculosis was perhaps the most important of these examples (see Figure 3.4). Popularly known as "consumption," tuberculosis probably killed more people than any other infectious disease at the end of the 19th century, having been attributed to one in seven deaths worldwide (Michael 1898). Even so, TB mortality had declined significantly by then, having achieved 57 per cent of its total reduction between 1838 and 1971 (McKeown 1976).

Effective biomedical treatments for TB were not available until the mid-20th century. The first antibiotic treatment for TB, streptomycin, was not prescribed until 1947, and the BCG vaccination was not made available until 1954. While medicines have since played a tremendous role in the prevention and treatment of tuberculosis, their contribution to the total decline since the previous century was surprisingly small. Assuming that TB would have continued its decline without antibiotics and vaccinations at the same rate before their appearance (1921–46), and generously assuming that antibiotics and immunization have reduced TB mortality by 50 per cent, then the contribution of these medicines to the decline between 1838 and 1971 would have been only about 3.2 per cent.

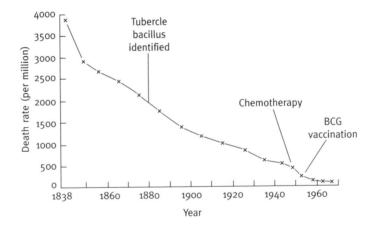

Figure 3.4. Mean annual death rates (standardized to 1901 population) for respiratory tuberculosis in England and Wales. It is striking to see that most of this decline occurred before the availability of effective anti-TB medications. McKeown, Thomas (1979). *The Role of Medicine: Dream, Mirage, or Nemesis.* Oxford: Basil Blackwell. p. 92. Reproduced with permission from John Wiley & Sons.

To be fair, McKeown acknowledges the role of biomedicine in some diseases. The smallpox vaccine had been available since the early 1800s, and it most likely played a major role in mortality decline, even before the collection of disease-specific statistics. Immunizations for typhus and tetanus, and antitoxin for diphtheria, also played important roles. But combined mortality for these diseases still comprised the minority of deaths for infectious diseases on the whole. Thus, the role of biomedicine in treating these diseases played only a minor role in the overall mortality decline of England and Wales. This conclusion is well established among medical historians and epidemiologists, including Omran, who reasonably extends it to other relatively affluent nations in his Classic Model (Omran 1971).

Having eliminated the role of biomedical technology, McKeown has us consider the relative efficacy of non-pharmacological measures. Despite a slight decline in the number of persons per residence in London, the overall trend toward urbanization during the Industrial Revolution would only have increased population density and its concomitant risks of disease transmission. Sanitation went from poor to worse as England's urban infrastructures failed to catch up with their expanding populations, resulting in problems like London cholera epidemics of 1849 and 1853–54 and the "Great Stink" of the River Thames in 1858 (Halliday 1999). Largely motivated by sanitary reformers such as Edwin Chadwick, England greatly improved its drinking water and waste-disposal systems in the late 1800s, but with the exception of some notable epidemics, water and food-borne diseases were already declining. As we saw earlier, cleaner obstetric methods greatly reduced childbirth fever in mothers and newborns, but these measures still only benefited a minority of the total population at risk for deadly infections.

McKeown cites a popular and oft-repeated quotation from one of Conan Doyle's Sherlock Holmes stories: "When we have eliminated the impossible, whatever remains, no matter how improbable, must be the truth." Having ruled out other major possibilities, McKeown identifies nutrition as the most prominent remaining factor, and thus, the primary determinant in the decline of infection-related mortality. Medical historians and social scientists often refer to this as the "McKeown Thesis."

McKeown offers three empirical arguments to support his thesis. The first is the well-known relationship between under-nutrition and infection. In Chapter 1, we reviewed some of the ways that different nutritional deficiencies impair certain mechanisms and structures of immune function. Tragically, there is no shortage of contemporary examples to demonstrate these relationships. The Food and Agriculture Organization (FAO) of the United Nations estimates that there are 825 million under-nourished people worldwide, and nearly one-third of all children in developing nations are under-nourished (Food and Agriculture Organization of the United Nations 2012). Under-nutrition is responsible for at least half of all child deaths each year, and more than half all deaths due to infectious pneumonias, diarrhea (i.e., gastrointestinal infections), malaria, and measles (Bryce et al. 2005). Combining our physiological understanding with these epidemiological data, it stands to reason that improved diets could have led to substantial improvements in child mortality in previous centuries—just as it *could* lead to substantial improvements in this century.

McKeown's second argument is that improved nutrition is the most likely common factor to explain the acceleration of population growth in different countries during the same time period. Such growth not only occurred in Europe and North America but also in countries such as Japan, Chile, and Sri Lanka (formerly known as Ceylon), societies that expanded under very different cultural and economic circumstances. Here, McKeown argues for a global increase in the availability and quality of food due to improved agricultural methods and transportation networks (1988). However, there is no direct evidence regarding overall food consumption during this period. Moreover, accelerated population growth began in most of these countries prior to their mortality declines. It is quite possible that these early expansions were artifacts of detection bias, as more people concentrated into urban areas, where they would have been more fully represented in national census statistics than their rural counterparts. Nevertheless, such artifacts would neither support nor refute the McKeown Thesis.

McKeown's third supporting argument harkens back to the lessons we learned from the First Epidemiological Transition. He correctly argues that the Agricultural Revolution led to the predominance of infectious diseases due to poor nutrition, poor sanitation, and crowding (although we would add social inequalities to this list). It follows that a change in one or more of these same human determinants would be responsible for the decline of infections 10 000 years later, especially in the absence of significant technological or bio-evolutionary changes. Once again, McKeown argues by elimination, ruling out improvements in sanitation and crowding in societies experiencing the early stages of industrialization. If anything, rapid urbanization during these periods exacerbated rather than improved these conditions, at least until the later decades of the 19th century (Burnett 1991). Among the major determinants of the First Transition, nutrition is the only remaining factor with the potential for historical improvement.

In addition to McKeown's arguments, population changes in body height and age of menarche (i.e., first menstruation) provide supporting evidence for nutrition as a major, if not primary, factor in the Second Epidemiological Transition. James Tanner, the pediatrician who developed the world's most widely used scales for childhood growth and development, maintains that such measures are mirrors of societal conditions. This is certainly the case for human stature, which has well-established links with nutritional status (Tanner 1992). It is therefore significant that many Second-Transition countries have seen secular (i.e., long-term) trends toward increasing stature in their adult populations, and that these trends coincide with major declines in infectious disease mortality. Such was the case for most European countries, which saw increases of 1–3 centimeters per decade in average adult heights during the second half of the 19th century (Cole 2000).

More recently, a study of thirty-one cohorts in ten European countries, as well as England and the United States, shows a significant correlation between height and childhood mortality, and more particularly, the mortality of infants between 28 days and 1 year of age (Bozzoli et al 2009). Most of these infant deaths are attributed to respiratory and gastrointestinal infections. It should also be noted that contemporary studies show significant correlations between infant birth weights and later growth as well as susceptibility to both infectious and chronic degenerative diseases (Barker 2007). Maternal stature is also correlated with birth weights, gestational growth, and pre-term births (Kramer 1998; Kramer et al. 1992). From parent to fetus, and from fetus to parent again, nutrition has long-lasting and profound effects on susceptibility to all manner of diseases across entire lifespans and multiple generations.

The age of menarche is a less direct but nevertheless sensitive indicator of nutritional status. This is especially evident in Scandanavian countries during the first half of the 20th century, when the mean age of menarche fell 12 months per decade until the Second World War (Cole 2000). These data are consistent with other European and North American countries, where the age of menarche fell from the late 19th to early 20th century (Euling et al. 2008). Interestingly, these trends also correlate with declining variability in the age of menarche. In Belgium, for instance, the oldest 10 percent of girls experiencing menarche declined the fastest while the youngest 10 percent hardly changed at all (Hauspie et al. 1997). These observations suggest that well-nourished populations may be reaching the lower age limits for menarche in our species. Indeed, the mean age of menarche appears to have stabilized in recent decades to around 12–13 years of age among the world's affluent societies. But more importantly, these observations also suggest that the reduction of inequalities can improve the health of entire populations, not just the least privileged within them. This is further supported by the reduction of variation in mortality rates between European countries during the same periods of mortality decline (Vallin 1991). The lesson here is that everyone, not just the poor, can benefit from an equitable distribution of resources for health and wellbeing.

3.3 McKeown's Critics and a Rejoinder

Nearly all health scholars agree that the biomedical fruit of Germ Theory played but a minor role in the decline of mortality in Europe and North America during the Industrial Revolution. Beyond this general agreement, however, some have criticized particular elements of the McKeown Thesis. One of these elements rests on the accuracy of diagnosis and related nosology (disease classification) used in 19th-century death records. One example was William Farr's standardized disease categories and the diagnostic criteria for determining causes of death in English mortality records, standards to which the General Register Office closely adhered until 1911 (Eyler 1979). Yet without belief in specific pathogens for infectious diseases, and little practical means for identifying such pathogens, physicians had to rely on potentially ambiguous diagnostic criteria. Even with the revolutionary medical technologies of the late 20th century, comparisons between antemortem diagnoses and the results of detailed autopsies in the same patients reveal error rates between 6 per cent and 68 per cent, with the worst rates for overlooked respiratory infections among the elderly (Gross et al. 1988).

Furthermore, it is difficult to attribute a primary cause of death when multiple and mutually interacting diseases are involved. Such is the case for today's syndemics. We previously discussed the syndemic nature of HIV, an immunodeficiency virus that renders the human host vulnerable to other infections, any of which might become the final cause of death. The same goes for the influenza virus, which is rarely the direct cause of flu-related deaths;

instead, the virus facilitates secondary bacterial infections of the lungs. It is for this reason that influenza was long thought to be a bacterial infection, and the namesake of *Hemophilis influenzae* (formerly, Pfeiffer's bacillus) turned out to be a misattribution (Crosby 1989). Noninfectious diseases can present even more of a problem. Adult onset diabetes is the chief determinant of kidney failure, and cardiovascular disease is the chief determinant of stroke—so which of these diseases should be put on a death certificate? With this dilemma in mind, it is not surprising that "heart failure" is one of the most common entries for cause of death among long-term care patients in the United States (Gross et al. 1988). After all, the heart usually stops by the time of the postmortem examination.

Others argue that McKeown underestimated the role of smallpox inoculation in the early years of mortality decline between the late 1700s and early 1800s (Mercer 1985). Even before Edward Jenner's discovery of *Vaccinia*, the English adopted a traditional Indian form of inoculation, known as variolation, that became popular after its use by the royal family in the 1740s. Until then, smallpox was endemic to major cities like London, where there were few if any gaps between major outbreaks in the first half of the 18th century. The London *Bills of Mortality* show significant declines in smallpox deaths in the later 1700s, around the same time as England's major population expansion. While causes of death for *Bills of Mortality* were commonly determined by people without medical training, full-blown cases of smallpox were easy enough to identify, and therefore, the data reliable enough for this particular disease.

That said, data for inoculation rates are incomplete or absent for England's many rural communities, just as they are for many of the world's affected countries at the time. In places like London, where such data exist, inoculation rates were far below the threshold required for the city's population to achieve what is known as "herd immunity:" the threshold at which enough people are immune to a disease such that it is more likely to die out than continue to spread (Mercer 1985).[2] Inoculation may indeed have played a role in protecting certain sub-populations against smallpox, but it is likely that patient isolation played an even greater role. There is a strong precedent for this in the final years of smallpox eradication, when epidemiologists from the US Centers for Disease Control (CDC) found themselves short of vaccines in West and Central Africa. Using a combination of patient isolation measures, and selective vaccination of direct contacts, the CDC team was able to control the spread of smallpox well below the threshold level needed to achieve herd immunity in these populations (Foege et al. 1975). It is possible that a similar combination of measures, deliberate or not, had a greater impact on smallpox mortality than Mckeown estimates.

Perhaps the more substantial criticism of the McKeown Thesis is that it places too much emphasis the role of nutrition over other non-medicinal factors. For instance, while McKeown correctly identifies poor housing conditions during the urban expansion of England up until

---

[2] Estimated herd immunity thresholds are based on the basic reproduction number (R_0) for a given disease—the average number of people infected for every single case, throughout the contagious period of the disease. The higher the basic reproduction number, the higher the estimated percentage for herd immunity.

the mid-1800s, many cities made significant housing improvements in later decades that correlated with steeper declines in infectious diseases (Burnett 1991). Building regulations set minimum room sizes, and large industrial cities such as Manchester placed outright bans on their notorious cellar dwellings. By 1885, the country had established twenty-eight Model Housing Trusts for working class families. Similar housing reforms were adopted on the European continent during the same period.

One could tell a similar story about the sanitary conditions of Europe's urban industrial environments. In 1848, Edwin Chadwick's *Report on the Labouring Populations of Great Britain* described the terrible stench of English cities, whose infrastructures lagged considerably behind their rapidly growing populations. Urban migration greatly increased the amount of solid waste that, along with the additional water of newly adopted flush toilets, overwhelmed city cesspools and treatment facilities such as they existed. Raw sewage spilled into rivers and groundwater, thereby contaminating drinking sources, and street drains that had originally been designed for rainwater became perpetual sewers for the output of factories and slaughterhouses. But as with urban housing, many English cities made significant improvements in waste disposal and drainage by the end of the 19th century, progress that was reflected, for example, in an 1896 survey of sanitary conditions in London and five other European capitals (Woods 1991).

McKeown may also have discounted the less technical contributions of professional health providers, especially with regard to basic sanitary reform practices. Miasma notwithstanding, North American and European countries adopted practices of improved nutrition, hygiene, and ventilation within increasingly standardized medical curricula. These practices, in turn, were further propagated with the expansion of home-health and visiting-nurse services in the early 20th century, such that professionals could teach and promote healthier living practices to families and communities while helping them to care for their sick (Kunitz 1991). Finally, in the interests of ventilation and rest, the isolation of infected patients may have greatly reduced the transmission of infectious diseases such as tuberculosis, for which many sanitaria were built. During the 1918 influenza pandemic, isolation measures were significantly correlated with disease mortality in US cities, some of which were hardly affected while others were devastated by the virus (Markel et al. 2007). Similarly, the addition of isolation measures probably aided in the eradication of smallpox in West and Central Africa at a time when there was not enough vaccine available (Fenner et al. 1988). As with the reduction in crowding, patient isolation measures can greatly reduce the sustainability of person-to-person disease transmission, even to the point that the rate of recovery outpaces the rate of new infections (Fenner et al. 1988).

It may be that the McKeown Thesis underestimates the contribution of these other non-medicinal factors to the decline of infectious disease mortality. Furthermore, it may be that different combinations of these factors may have contributed more than nutrition to declines within certain societies and certain historical moments. But these relative differences do not detract from the chief lesson of the Second Epidemiological Transition: that the sum total of these lifestyle factors is largely responsible for the first major decline of infectious diseases since they first emerged with agriculture in the Neolithic.

Comparing the Agricultural Revolution with the Industrial Revolution, we find the same human determinants of infectious disease: a) subsistence, via its affects on nutritional status and immunity; b) settlement, via its effects on population density, living conditions, and sanitation; and, c) social organization, via the distributions of these resources and their differences within and between groups. In the earlier case, poor diets, crowded living, and social inequalities created selective conditions for the emergence of acute infectious diseases. In the later case, improved diets, reduced crowding, and a broader distribution of resources across social classes created conditions for the decline of these same infections. As such, the First and Second Transition could be seen as two sides of the same epidemiological coin with human actions as the basic currency.

3.4 Health Trade-offs and the Shape of Things to Come

The Second Epidemiological Transition brought substantial increases in life expectancy among the affluent societies of the industrialized world. Averaging the seven countries that began the Second Transition before 1880, life expectancy at birth increased by more than 85 per cent from the beginning to end of the 20th century (Riley 2005). These statistics certainly reflect dramatic improvements in human health, but it should be noted that life expectancy is a strange kind of average, one that is calculated based on the probabilities of people at each age surviving to their next age during a given year. That said, a subsequent improvement in life expectancy does mean that more people of different ages are living longer. In the case of the Second Epidemiological Transition, more people were surviving infectious diseases in childhood, and because of this, more people had an opportunity to grow old.

With more people living to older ages, the Second Transition brought certain health trade-offs, the most important being a shift from acute infections to chronic non-infectious diseases as the primary causes of death. Then as now, these so-called "diseases of civilization" included cancer, diabetes, coronary artery disease, and the chronic obstructive pulmonary diseases of emphysema and asthma (Barrett et al. 1998). To some extent, we can attribute these diseases to the aging process. For instance, nearly all forms of cancer result from mutations in genes responsible for the regulation of cell growth and differentiation. In the absence of regulation, cells can proliferate out of control. Unless these cells are checked by the immune system, or somehow die on their own, then they will continue to grow and spread until they disrupt major organ systems. Even for the healthiest among us, every natural cell division is a role of the dice that carries some risk for one of these cancer-causing mutations. And every year of life increases this risk with additional rolls of the dice. Likewise for heart disease, even healthy individuals will accumulate plaque in their arteries and their cardiac output will continue to decrease after 35 years of age. We are all mortal, and we all have to die of something.

Aging aside, industrialization contributed to the rise of chronic disease through artificial living environments. Particularly in urban environments, water and air pollution has been linked to significantly higher rates of cancer, birth defects, allergies, and impeded mental development (Andrade et al. 2012; Asher 2011; Ebenstein 2012; van der Linde et al. 2011). These issues are compounded by the stresses of urbanization, which are correlated with increased levels and incidences of hypertension, as well as depression and anxiety (Galea 2011; Huang et al. 2010). In turn, these psychological effects are closely linked with high-risk behaviors such as smoking, drug and alcohol use, violence, and unsafe sexual practices. Finally, all these risks are inversely correlated with socio-economic status and are often experienced very differently according to gender, ethnicity, and people's conceptions of race.[3] Buried within national statistics, the poorest people of the richest countries continue to experience the highest morbidity and mortality as diseases of civilization become diseases of poverty.

We began this book with the pronouncements of health authorities declaring the end of all human infections and calling for a primary focus on chronic diseases. These pronouncements are at least somewhat understandable given the major health shifts of the Second Epidemiological Transition. But as we will see, the Second Transition was experienced very differently in poor nations, just as it was for the poorest communities of rich nations. Adding to this global problem, the aging of world populations and the rise of chronic diseases have created new syndemics of infectious and non-infectious diseases, as well as new reservoirs for the transmission of novel, virulent, and drug-resistant pathogens.

[3] Race is not a useful biological category due to the gradations of human variation, the independence of heritable traits, and the fact that there is more variation within human groups than between them. That said, anthropologists recognize that race is still highly relevant as a social category (Brown and Armelagos 2001).

4

The Worst of Both Worlds

We live in a world where infections pass easily across borders—social and geographic—while resources, including cumulative scientific knowledge, are blocked at customs.
Social Inequalities and Emerging Infectious Diseases. Paul Farmer (1996)

Thus far, we have examined the Classic Model of the Second Epidemiological Transition, which is based on the experience of a few affluent nations in the industrialized world. Encouraged by these examples, many public health authorities of the 1970s and 1980s hoped that poorer nations of the world would achieve similar health improvements once they became sufficiently industrialized, and that this would lead to the eradication of most infectious diseases by the beginning of the 20th century. Instead, the Second Transition was experienced very differently among poorer societies, many of whom did not begin their shifts until after the Second World War. Despite rapid initial gains, most of these late mortality declines turned out to be more modest than those in wealthier countries.

At the same time, the developing world saw substantial increases in chronic degenerative diseases. Rapid urbanization in poor countries brought steep fertility declines, which resulted in increasingly aging populations. While affluent nations continue to have higher percentages of older people than their poorer counterparts, more than half the world's elderly live in poor nations with insufficient resources to care for them (Kinsella and Velkoff 2001). Finally, the late mortality declines of poor countries have been much more dependent on antimicrobial medicines than the changing living standards of richer countries in the Classic Model. Given the increasing prevalence of drug-resistant infections, such dependence bodes ill for the future of global health.

Considering these factors in combination, we see the emergence of a worst-of-both-worlds scenario: an incomplete Second Transition with too many remaining infections and greater opportunities for syndemics with chronic diseases (cf. Bradley 1993). Here, the elderly poor represent a growing reservoir for new infections, and heavy dependence on antibiotics is further accelerating the evolution of drug resistance. Under these conditions, the Classic Model of the Second Transition is not sustainable in the developing world. Given the porous nature of international borders, it will only be a matter of time before historical infections came back to haunt the wealthier nations of the world—a so-called "re-emergence" of infectious diseases that diminished but never fully disappeared.

An Unnatural History of Emerging Infections. First Edition. Ron Barrett and George J. Armelagos
© Ron Barrett and George J. Armelagos 2013. Published 2013 by Oxford University Press.

4.1 Delayed and Incomplete Transitions

There are 119 countries for which we have enough data to identify a beginning point for the Second Epidemiological Transition (Riley 2005). Among these, only seven nations began their transition before 1850, and another seventeen before 1900. Except for the inclusion of Mexico and Japan, this group represented the wealthiest nations of Western Europe and its former colonies. The next major cluster of transitions occurred in the interwar period of the 1920s and 1930s, affecting the less developed, (sometimes known as "second world") nations of Latin America, Eastern and Southern Europe, and a few nations in Asia and Africa. Almost all the remaining transitions occurred after the Second World War (see Figure 4.1). These later declines comprised most of the Second Epidemiological Transition, affecting the large majority of the total human population. In 1875, about 10.5 per cent of the human population was undergoing the Second Transition; by 1960, the figure increased to 96.4 per cent due to the addition of these later transitions. By including these poorer, late-transitioning societies, the estimated worldwide life expectancy at birth increased by more than ten years in the next four decades: from 52 years in 1963, to 66 years in 2003 (Bloom and Canning 2007).

Yet despite impressive gains, the delayed transitions of the developing world masked important differences within and between societies. To begin with, Second Transition societies continued to group into two different clusters, which could be described as "convergence clubs" (Mayer-Foulkes 2001). The "low mortality club" consisted of richer nations whose life expectancies converged at around 75 years at the turn of the Millennium. The "high mortality club" consisted of poorer nations whose life expectancies converged at the same time at around 50 years of age. While a few poorer nations, such as Costa Rica, made the jump from high to low mortality during the decades leading up to the 21st century, most of the developing world remained in the high mortality club (Bloom and Canning 2007).

An optimist might still predict that it is only a matter of time before the rest of the developing world catches up and joins the low mortality club. After all, most low mortality countries were those who began the Second Transition much earlier and thus had more time to reach healthier levels of life expectancy. Indeed, many late-transition societies made very rapid gains in their initial years of their Second Transition, with rates of improvement that could have caught up with the health of low mortality nations. But instead, a number of these nations slowed down and then leveled off their mortality improvements. Others have since fallen into a "mortality trap," regressing from earlier improvements, either because of political turmoil such as civil wars, genocide, the fall of the Soviet Union, or because of the emergence of HIV/AIDS, especially in the poorest societies of sub-Saharan Africa (Soares 2007).

Significantly, the human determinants of the Second Transition have been different for economically under-developed societies than for their well-developed counterparts. Among the latter, life expectancies have been positively correlated with economic indicators such as per capita income level and gross domestic product (GDP). In contrast, many health improvements in the developing world have occurred despite little if any gains in GDP, and in some countries, they have occurred in the face of declining economic conditions (Soares 2007).

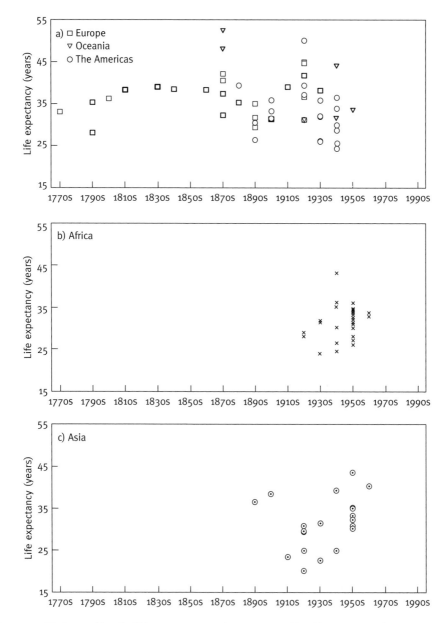

Figure 4.1. Timing and level of life expectancy at the initiation of health transitions (plotted by period of initiation). Note that only seven countries began the Second Transition before the early 1800s. Most developing countries began the transition after the Second World War. Riley J. C. (2005). The Timing and Pace of Health Transitions around the World. *Population and Development Review*. 31(4): 744. Reproduced with permission from John Wiley & Sons.

This is not to say that economic improvement is unimportant for health improvement. On the contrary, the unsustainable and often temporary nature of health improvements in perpetually impoverished societies underscores the importance of economic development, especially as it pertains to the equitable distribution of material resources for human wellbeing.

From the end of the Second World War, vaccines and antibiotics have increasingly served as buffers against the health effects of inadequate living conditions among poor societies of the world. Insofar as they addressed respiratory and gastrointestinal infections, these medicines were responsible for more than 50 per cent of the mortality declines in developing nations up through the late 1970s (Preston 1980). Depending on the geographic region, the implementation of antimalarial drugs and DDT spraying reduced mortality by another 13–33 per cent during the same time period. But these declines did not contribute as much to the reduction of child mortality as they did in the previous one hundred years (Soares 2007). As in centuries past, respiratory and gastrointestinal infections continued to be the main causes of death for children under 5 years of age in the developing world. This should not be surprising as the majority of the world's population continued to live in poverty, without secure food resources, and crowded into unsanitary dwellings. Despite the miracles of modern medicine, the conditions that brought about the First Transition persisted into the final decades of the Second Transition. As we will see in the Chapter 6, it would only be a matter of time before drug-resistant pathogens would begin removing these medicinal buffers and the infections of poverty would re-emerge and spread through an increasingly global human disease ecology.

4.2 Chronic Diseases and New Syndemics

In many cases, the limited and transient nature of declining infections in developing societies has not impeded the rise of non-contagious diseases, such as cancer, heart disease, and diabetes, which are classically associated with the Second Epidemiological Transition. By the turn of the Millennium, chronic disease mortality surpassed infectious disease mortality in all continents except Africa (Kanavos 2006). Chronic diseases are especially prevalent in historically poor populations transitioning from localized subsistence agriculture to large-scale agribusiness. Within these societies, chronic diseases often appear first in the upper socioeconomic classes because of their greater access to Western products such as industrially processed foods (Armelagos et al. 2005). But these foods soon "trickle down" to the poorest classes as they become more affordable and available than healthier alternatives. As such, many people cannot afford to purchase food that meets their nutritional requirements.

Barry Popkin coined the term "nutrition transition" to describe the dietary changes that have resulted from the globalization of industrial food production (1994). These changes have brought increasing prevalences of obesity, cardiovascular disease, cerebrovascular disease, and adult onset diabetes in developing nations. For example, India is experiencing a major epidemic of adult onset diabetes, with 20 million estimated cases expected to increase by more than 150 per cent over the next two decades (Green et al. 2002). Yet despite recent economic gains, India faces the challenges other developing nations face, and it can ill afford the additional burden of heart disease, stroke, kidney failure, amputations, and blindness associated with this disease.

In addition to direct health consequences, the chronic diseases can have syndemic relationships with major infectious diseases. Diabetes has long been linked to increased TB susceptibility and mortality (Root 1934). One study in Tanzania found that subjects with an impaired glucose test were four times more likely to contract tuberculosis (Mugusi et al. 1990). A nearly sevenfold increase in the risk for TB infection among Type 2 diabetes patients in southern Mexico is comparable to HIV patients in the same area (Ponce-De-Leon et al. 2004). Similar dynamics can be found in China, where diabetes and heart disease significantly increased the risk of death for infected patients during the SARS epidemic (Chan et al. 2003).

Cancer has also had substantial impacts, both direct and syndemic, on late-transitioning societies of the developing world. In 2008, cancer in under-developed nations accounted for 56 per cent of the 12.7 million reported cases worldwide. It also accounted for 64 per cent of the 7.4 million deaths, having risen to become the second leading cause of mortality in the poorer societies of the world (Jemal et al. 2011). As with the affluent world, breast cancer is the most frequently diagnosed cancer and leading cause of cancer-related deaths among females while lung cancer leads among males in frequency and cause of cancer-related deaths. But because of late detection and the unavailability of many chemotherapeutic agents, the mortality rates for these and other cancers is much higher in poor societies, often more than 80 per cent for otherwise treatable tumors.

In addition, infectious diseases are more likely to cause cancers in developing societies. Whereas only 10 per cent of cancers in affluent nations are attributable to infectious diseases, that proportion increases to more than 25 per cent in underdeveloped nations (Kanavos 2006). The human papilloma virus (HPV) has been linked to similar rates of cervical and colorectal cancers in both affluent and poor nations, but the rate of malignancies is five times greater among the latter. There is also a list of HIV-related cancers caused by other viruses such as Kaposi's sarcoma (HHV8) and non-Hodgkin's lymphoma (EBV). Food-borne and water-borne infections caused by *Heliobacter pylori* are associated with a two to threefold increased risk for stomach cancers, which are unusually prevalent in the developing countries of Latin America.

Finally, the well-known association between cancer and pollution should be examined in the context of urbanization in the developing world. Since the end of the 20th century, the majority of the world's human population lives in urban environments (World Resources 1996). But in developing societies these environments are often subject to much higher levels of vehicular and industrial pollution than the cities of well-developed societies. This is often because industrialization occurs at a much faster pace than infrastructural development in poor societies. It is also often because of poor environmental regulation in many of these societies, a situation that is commonly exploited by multinational corporations seeking to outsource their waste-generating activities—a practice known as "dumping" (Patz et al. 1996). Not surprisingly, many of the world's most hazardous factories are located near urban slums with large cancer clusters in their populations.

4.3 Aging and Poverty

More than half the world's people over 65 years of age live in developing countries, and the elderly poor are expected to account for most of a projected increase from 460 million people in 1990 to 1.4 billion in 2030 (Kinsella and Velkoff 2001). Part of this increase stems from greater survival to adulthood among late Second Transition societies, which has improved the odds of their members living into older years. But the increased proportion of elderly in these populations is also due to the "baby busts" that usually accompany the urbanization of large populations. Demographers use population pyramids to illustrate this kind of change in the proportion of people at different ages, also known as the age structure of a population.

Figure 4.2 shows three population pyramids representing different age structures for the world population at three time periods. Each of these pyramids consists of two bar graphs (histograms) that have been turned on their sides and placed beside each other to depict the relative numbers of males and females in five-year age increments: from 0–5 years of age at the bottom, to 80+ years of age at the top. Each of these pyramids is essentially two pyramids: a darker interior pyramid representing the combined age structures of developed nations, and a lighter exterior pyramid representing those of developing nations. The 1950 pyramid is fairly triangular for developed and developing nations alike. The 1990 pyramid depicts the middle bulge of the adult "baby boomers" in developed nations, but maintains the triangular shape of relatively young populations in the developing world due to later mortality declines.

By 2030, the pyramid is projected to bulge into a columnar, or beehive appearance in both its dark and light portions, reflecting the aging populations of developed and developing nations respectively. But the similarity of the trends masks at least two important differences. First, the aging of poorer societies has been largely driven by baby busts that accompanied the rapid urbanization of the developing world. Some of these busts can be attributed to successful and sometimes controversial family planning programs. But many others can be attributed to rapid urbanization and rural-to-urban migration, which has led to steep fertility declines as large families became more costly, economic mobility became more important, and children were no longer needed for agricultural labor. This has resulted in a kinship transition involving the contraction of traditional extended families, their fragmentation into nuclear subunits, and finally, their geographic dispersion, either due to the "push factors" of economic hardship, or the "pull factors" of economic opportunity.

The second important difference concerns the health and economic impacts of dependency among the frail elderly, which are more acutely felt in poor societies. Healthy older and third generation family members are often important assets for households, having the potential to make contributions in childcare or economic activities. But frail elderly present an additional challenge for the second generation of working adults who must then care for their parents and children simultaneously. This is challenge enough for families in affluent societies, whose working adults have come to be known as the "sandwich generation." The challenge is all the more difficult in the sandwich generations of poor societies, who often

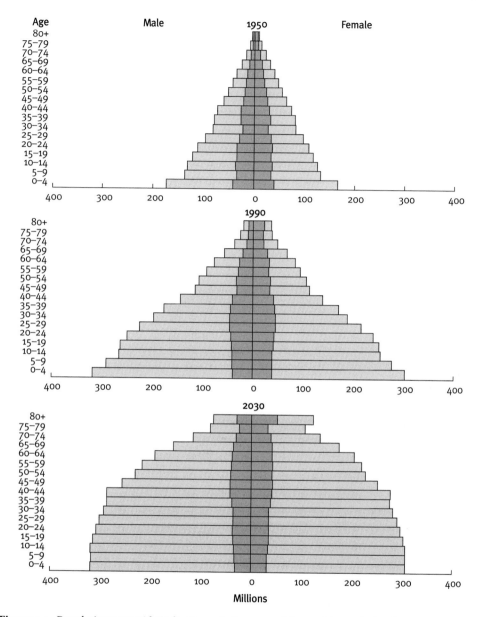

Figure 4.2. Population pyramids indicating relative ages of the world population by sex in 1950 and 1990, and a population estimate for 2030. The darker colors indicate developed nations. The lighter colors represent developing nations. Most societies, both rich and poor, are trending toward bulging pyramids with aging populations. Kinsella, A. and V.A. Velkoff 2001. *An Aging World: 2001.* Washington D.C.: U.S. Census Bureau.

face the double bind of diminished financial resources and diminishing social supports from scattered and shrinking family support networks.

These challenges come to the fore when older members of poor societies become sick. Under these circumstances, impoverished families face difficult decisions about the allocation of resources: whether to pay for medicines versus food, a clinic visit versus a pair of shoes, or another hospitalization versus another year of school fees. Compounding these dilemmas, the indirect costs of an illness are often higher than the direct costs. This is especially the case when working family members must forgo wage-earning labor to accompany a sick parent on long journeys to health providers or long waits in overcrowded clinics. Many hospitals in developing countries expect accompanying family members to provide meals and basic care such as bathing, laundry, and even routine administration of medications (cf. Barrett 2008). All of this can add up to days of missed wages for families surviving on narrow economic margins.

Faced with these expenses, it is not uncommon for impoverished families to forgo, delay, or otherwise compromise the medical treatment of their elderly members. Such decisions may be reinforced by historical expectations about when and how elderly people are supposed to die. For instance, North Americans once referred to pneumonia as the "old man's friend," with the idea that it was a relatively quick and painless way to die for people who did not usually live much beyond 65 years. But respiratory infections, such as influenza and tuberculosis, most often affect both the very young and the very old in U-shaped curves of infection by age. Consequently, higher rates of infection among the elderly can greatly increase the risk of infection among young children. In this manner, the "old man's friend" can quickly become the poor child's enemy.

As with the increase of chronic degenerative diseases, the aging of the developing world has created unwilling reservoirs for the evolution of virulent and drug resistant infections. A very good example of this can be found in the relationship between seasonal and pandemic influenzas. Seasonal influenza viruses, such as the H2N2 and H3N2 strains, infect and kill a disproportionate number of elderly every year, and they will do so increasingly with the aging of the world's populations (Thompson et al. 2006). Even more alarming, the size of seasonal influenza epidemics contributes to the yearly antigenic variation of the virus, and hence, to the probability of emerging pathogenic strains, such as the H5N1 avian influenzas and the H1N1 swine influenza of the early 21st century (Boni et al. 2004). Thus, increasing rates of seasonal influenza among the elderly increases the probability of pandemic influenza in people of all ages.

Recall that influenza-related deaths are usually caused by secondary bacterial pneumonias. There is experimental evidence that persons with pre-existing respiratory infections can become super-spreaders for secondary infections, the so-called "cloud effect," which has been observed in the dissemination of methicillin-resistant *Staph. aureus* (MRSA) as well as the coronavirus associated with severe acute respiratory syndrome (SARS), a recently discovered infection from which the elderly were more likely to die (Sherertz et al. 1996; Chan et al. 2003) (see Figure 4.3).

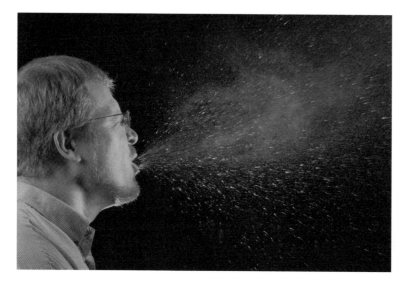

Figure 4.3. Sneeze in progress, depicting a cone-shaped plume of respiratory droplets being expelled from the nose and mouth. People with additional respiratory conditions can sometimes transmit a pathogen further than if they were infected by one disease alone. This is sometimes referred to as the "cloud effect." Photograph by Brian Judd. U.S. Centers for Disease Control and Prevention.

In addition, elderly populations have often served as reservoirs for antibiotic resistance in bacterial pathogens such as *Staphylococcus aureus, Pseudomonas auregenosa*, and *Klebsiella pneumoniae*, which have become endemic to nursing homes and long-term care facilities in the United Kingdom and North America (Smith et al. 2000). Although nursing homes are beginning to appear in larger cities of the developing world, they are still quite rare in non-Western societies. More common is the inappropriate and incomplete use of antibiotics, which is especially prevalent in developing countries where low-cost generic medicines can be readily obtained without prescriptions. Such medicines present cheap alternatives to professional medical care when older people become sick in poor societies. As we will see later, such practices have greatly contributed to the evolution of drug-resistant pathogens.

4.4 Accelerated Globalization and Re-emerging Awareness

Epidemiologists have used a fire analogy to describe the behavior of infectious diseases. Like fires, infections spread from neighbor to neighbor. Like fires, infections are more likely to emerge in vulnerable communities. And like fires, infections can sometimes spread out of control, affecting all communities, no matter how well protected they might otherwise be.

Now imagine if your local fire department only protected some houses in your neighborhood and not others. Your house is protected, but your neighbor's house is not. One day, a fire breaks out in your neighbor's house. With no access to professional firefighters, your neighbor's fire continues to burn until it ignites *your* house. Even if your fire department extinguishes the fire in a timely manner, which it may not, the damage to your home would still be worse than if it had never caught fire in the first place. Furthermore, your risk of future fires would remain elevated until the fire department protected everyone in your neighborhood. Such is the case of infectious diseases, for which the accelerated pace of globalization has transformed the world of potential human hosts into a highly connected neighborhood.

The recent history of smallpox presents an excellent case in point. By the mid-20th century, smallpox had been all but eliminated in affluent Western societies. But the virus persisted in other parts of the world, especially in the poorer societies of Asia and sub-Saharan Africa. Because of this, Europe and North America experienced continued to have limited, "re-importation epidemics" from the end of the Second World War to the final eradication of the disease in 1980 (Barrett 2006a). During this period, no one was completely safe until everyone was completely safe from the disease.

The same example makes the case in fiscal terms. Barring the unlikely event of a bioterrorist attack, current annual expenditures for smallpox prevention is US$0.00 in the United States, €0.00 in Europe, ¥0.00 in Japan, and so forth. The same could not be said for polio prevention, for which the US alone has spent US$35 billion on vaccinations from 1955–2005 (Thompson et al. 2006). As with smallpox prevention, all this money could be saved with the worldwide eradication of polio. We hope that most people do not think about health matters in purely fiscal terms. But for those who do, the globalization of infectious diseases makes a powerful and pragmatic case against isolationism.

As we know from Chapter 2, the globalization of human networks has been occurring for quite a long time. By 2000 BCE, irrigation agriculture had spread throughout the Eurasian continents, and with it came the rise of many state level societies. By 500 BCE, the majority of inhabited Eurasian land was under some form of state control, and many of these states were linked by extensive trade networks that stretched from the Mediterranean to the Yangstze River (McNeill 1976). People, goods, and animals moved along these networks, in times of war and of peace, and with them flowed the viruses, bacteria, and parasites that brought the acute infections of the First Transition. From Columbus ill-fated landing in 1492, these infections rapidly spread from the Old World to the New World. For the next four centuries, the sun never set on the First Epidemiological Transition.

The health gains of the Second Transition did not spread so fast. From its early emergence in the late 18th century, infectious disease mortality had been declining in seven nations over eighty years before it declined elsewhere, and at least another one hundred years before it began declining in poorer nations of the developing world. Even then, these declines were more modest and limited in under-developed societies in comparison with their affluent counterparts. At the same time, many poor nations experienced rapid increases in chronic diseases within rapidly aging populations, creating new reservoirs and new syndemics for infectious diseases. While health authorities of the affluent world were predicting the end of human infections, the rest of the world was still dealing with old problems that had never been fully addressed. At a global level, human infections had been partly submerged rather than eradicated. With the human world transformed into a single neighborhood, it was only a matter of time before these problems re-emerged to haunt societies both rich and poor. The remedies of the Second Transition came too little and too late.

The pace of globalization has accelerated exponentially since the Second Transition first began. From 1800 to the present day, human mobility has increased more than a thousand-fold in industrial societies (Saker et al. 2004). Much of this is due to the advent and increasing availability of commercial air transport in the 20th century. The number of commercial air passengers has increased 8 to 9 per cent nearly every year since 1960. At any given moment, there are at least 50 000 commercial passenger planes in the air; these carry more than 1.5 billion people a year, of whom more than 700 million are international travelers (MacPherson et al. 2009) (see Figure 4.4).

Consider the speed of all this air travel in relation to the clinical course of infectious diseases. Back in the days of steamships, a transatlantic voyage took about ten days; as such, a traveller who had been newly infected with *Vibro cholera* would run the course of the disease weeks before reaching port. During a typhus fever epidemic in the 1890s, newly arrived immigrants to Ellis Island who were infected usually presented signs of the disease before completing the entry process (Markel 2003). But with air transport, even a pathogenic virus with a fast incubation period could be carried by an unwitting traveler to the other side of the globe, and transmitted to other travelers in the interim, well before the first signs of the disease appeared.

A good example of this occurred in 2007, when Andrew Speaker, a personal injury attorney from the United States, chose to take an international vacation despite having a positive culture for extremely drug-resistant tuberculosis (XDR TB)—a highly virulent and dangerous form of the infection (McGee 2007). Speaker, who was asymptomatic for the disease, travelled

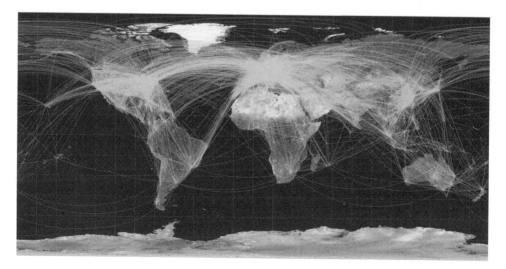

Figure 4.4. World map of airline routes in 2009. This map depicts 54 317 official routes. There are 50 000 commercial airplanes in the air at any given moment. Jpatokal 2009. Creative Commons Attribution Share Alike 3.0.

in seven airplanes over twelve days, visiting Paris, Athens, two Greek Islands, Rome, Prague, and Montreal before returning to his home town of Atlanta, where his father-in-law worked as a microbiologist for the CDC. During the interim period, Mr Speaker could have infected up to 1280 of his fellow international passengers, and many more travelers and locals in the five countries he visited. Fortunately, Mr. Speaker never came down with the full-blown disease, nor did his known contacts. But the consequences could have been severe and far-reaching.

Adding to the challenges of rapid air travel, another 1 billion people travel long distances each year over land and water (MacPherson et al. 2009). It is estimated that 175 million people live outside their country of birth and that there are 81 million migrant laborers globally. This does not include another 50 million internally displaced people and nearly 20 million international refugees in the world. The latter groups are especially prone to outbreaks of virulent and drug resistant forms of cholera, plague, and tuberculosis. Given the connections between these populations and the rest of the world, it is no longer safe to say these problems only affect (or infect) those in poor, exotic, and far-away places. Everyone is our neighbor these days. Everyone lives only a few hours away from us. When it comes to infectious diseases, everyone's problems increase the risk that anyone else will have the same problems.

Explaining why she never returned to her home town, Gertrude Stein famously said "there is no there there." With the globalization of human societies, we could turn the phrase to say "there is no there here." Humankind is rapidly developing a single, global disease ecology, one that involves the convergence of chronic and infectious diseases as well as the diffusion of pathogens across social and national boundaries. This convergence represents a Third Epidemiologic Transition, characterized by the evolution of human transmissibility, human virulence, and antimicrobial resistance of infectious pathogens. Applying the lessons learned thus far, we will henceforth devote the remainder of this book to a critical examination of the Third Transition.

Part Three

The Third Transition

5

New Diseases, Raw and Cooked

Examining the human determinants of avian influenzas, Mike Davis, an urban theorist and historian, states that "the superurbanization of the human population...has been paralleled by an equally dense urbanization of its meat supply." He then asks, "Could production density become a synonym of viral density?" (Davis 2006: 84). We believe it could, but that humans also engage in other large-scale and far-reaching practices that increase our exposure to non-human (i.e., raw) pathogens and domesticate them into human (i.e., cooked) varieties.

Our story begins in March of 2003, when one of us (Barrett) traveled through Hong Kong only three days after the international news media reported a new infectious disease outbreak in China. Researchers had yet to identify the microbe responsible for this novel infection, but they had already given it a label: Severe Acute Respiratory Syndrome (SARS). True to its name, SARS was highly virulent; it would ultimately kill 774 people out of more than 8 000 reported cases (Anderson et al. 2004). The infection was also rapidly spreading across international borders, with cases reported on mainland China, in Vietnam, Singapore, and Canada. It appeared from these early signs that SARS could become a deadly pandemic (cf. Kleinman and Watson 2005).

Barrett narrates his experience:

Arriving at the Hong Kong airport, I was immediately greeted by masked public health workers, who inquired about my health while taking my temperature with a thermal scanner on my forehead. Having been medically cleared, I proceeded on through the airport and spent the day in the major island of the city while waiting for an onward flight to India later that evening. I noticed the streets were less busy than usual, and many of the wet market venders had closed their shops. Normally, a visitor could spend hours trying to identify all the sea creatures being sold for human consumption. But not on this day.

All around me, people were wearing scarves and makeshift masks over their mouths and noses. I was not among them, knowing that nothing short of a proper filtration mask would protect against the inhalation or expulsion of pathogen-laden respiratory micro-droplets. Indeed, the makeshift masks often make matters worse, becoming moist platforms for all manner of respiratory infections. Yet when I returned from India to Hong Kong two weeks later, not only were the cloth masks more popular than ever, but many were designer masks, well co-ordinated with urban business attire. Fashion had caught up with the SARS epidemic, even if public health had not.

Following Barrett's return to the US, we were both teaching emerging infections courses at our respective universities. The new SARS epidemic gave us an opportunity to discuss the human determinants of emerging infections, and we did so with a series of predictions.

An Unnatural History of Emerging Infections. First Edition. Ron Barrett and George J. Armelagos.
© Ron Barrett and George J. Armelagos 2013. Published 2013 by Oxford University Press.

1. The pathogen will have a zoonotic origin; one or more nonhuman species to which it is much better adapted than it is to humans.
2. Transmission to humans will be linked to environmental encroachment into wild animal habitats and/or the handling of host animals for market-based food consumption.
3. Transmission among humans will be highest in the most densely populated areas.
4. Transmission among humans will mainly occur through food, water, and hand-to-mouth contact.

Classroom theater notwithstanding, these predictions were not as premonitory as they appeared. Most newly identified human pathogens have zoonotic origins, and the SARS corona virus (CoV) is no exception. The virus was initially detected in civet cats that were being sold in wet markets of the Guangdong Province, but phylogenic comparisons of different corona virus variants strongly suggest that Horseshoe bats are the main host, and that these animals may have infected nearby civets while they too were being sold at the wet markets (Lau et al. 2005). Either way, exposure to the virus was facilitated by the hunting and capture of wild animals for sale as exotic foods or as ingredients for cosmetics, perfumes, or traditional Chinese medicines.

Our classes examined the relationship between disease transmission and population density that we discussed in previous chapters. To illustrate this point, one of us had used an image from Hong Kong's Amoy Gardens well before the SARS outbreak. With over 50 000 people per square kilometer, Amoy Gardens is located in one of the world's most densely populated districts. The apartments themselves are a testament to dense urban living, with nineteen tightly packed thirty-three-storey residential buildings. Unfortunately, Amoy Gardens also became the site of the densest SARS cluster of the 2002–3 epidemic, with 329 confirmed cases and forty-two deaths (Lee et al. 2005). Wipe tests indicated that the virus had been transmitted via contaminated water, which had back-flowed from the sewage system and up through the floor drains in neighboring bathrooms. The water was then scattered by bathroom ventilation fans, landing on counters and fixtures that could then be touched by human hands (McKinney et al. 2006). At Amoy Gardens, SARS had spread via bad plumbing throughout the building, and then via hand-to-mouth throughout the community.

The 2002–3 SARS epidemic illustrates how the same major determinants of emerging infections in the First Transition have helped to bring new infections into 21st-century populations. Subsistence practices brought humans into contact with infected animals. Settlement patterns squeezed susceptible host populations into cities and stacked them in skyscrapers with poor plumbing. Certain forms of social organization produced inequalities such that some people needed to hunt exotic wild animals for food and money, and some people had to live in dense and sometimes dangerous environments. Add to this the demographic and health changes of the Second Transition, such that the majority of SARS-related deaths occurred among people over 60 years of age, and people with pre-existing chronic diseases were more likely to contract and spread the disease, just as they were more likely to die from it. Combine these factors and we have the makings of the Third Epidemiological Transition.

In this chapter, we examine three closely related features of acute human infections in the Third Epidemiological Transition. The first is the entry of new pathogens into the human population. Like SARS, most of these new infections evolved from zoonotic infections that first entered the human population in "raw" forms that made them difficult to transmit from human to human. We then examine the conditions in which these "raw" diseases become "cooked"—how they adapt to human populations in such a way that they are capable of sustained human-to-human transmission. Finally, we examine the evolution of virulence among these pathogens: the ways they make us very sick, or only a little sick, and their strategies for doing so. As we will see, the evolutionary dynamics of these pathogens can have some surprising twists. Nevertheless, the selective conditions for their evolution are more straightforward. No matter how great or "revolutionary" our activities may be, they still boil down to three basic categories of human health determinants: subsistence, settlement, and social organization.

5.1 The Evolution of Invasion

Epidemiologists have discovered 335 novel human pathogens between 1940 and 2004, and the number of these discoveries significantly increased after 1980 (Jones et al. 2008).[1] As we mentioned in the introduction, it is possible that some of these pathogens had been circulating among people for some time before their discovery, becoming "newly identified" as a result of recently improved detection methods. Affluent societies are especially prone to this kind of detection bias because they usually have better developed disease surveillance systems. Consequently, they are often the first to report new infections even if later studies reveal earlier entry into poor societies. Yet regardless of delays and biases, phylogenetic comparisons of newly identified strains indicate that most of these pathogens are indeed new invaders of the human species. We must therefore examine the evolutionary conditions in which these invasions occur.

Although many pathogens may be newly emerging, the selective conditions for their emergence are as old as the Neolithic. Then as now, most new infections arose from zoonotic infections, which then evolved human transmissibility as we changed our modes of subsistence and thus changed our relationships with other animal host species. During the Neolithic, the domestication of animals created new opportunities for zoonotic infections to "make the jump" into human host populations. Today, the human exploitation of wild species, encroachment onto new environments, and industrialization of food production (especially meat) have created more opportunities for these infections to jump from animal to human. The scales of these changes are much larger, and their speeds much faster, than they were in the Neolithic, but the determining role of human subsistence remains the same.

Most newly identified pathogens originated as zoonotic infections of wild or domesticated animal species. Among the 335 novel infections discussed above, more than 60 per cent originated in nonhuman animal species, among which 70 per cent were wild animal populations (Jones et al. 2008). Given the thousands of years that humans have been living with

---

[1] It should be noted that the number of newly identified pathogens declined after 1990 but still remained higher than all other decades before 1980.

domesticated animals and acquiring their diseases, it makes sense that most of our new zoonotic origin infections would arise from wild animals with whom we had less contact. But this does not explain why the number of novel human infections has increased in recent decades. To understand this, we must take a closer look our changing relationships to specific groups of animals and their environments.

Nonhuman primates are a major source of human infections both new and old. While nonhuman primates constitute about 0.5 per cent of all vertebrate species, they have been the earlier hosts and ongoing reservoirs of more than 20 per cent of all human infections (Wolfe et al. 2007). These include new infections such as HIV, Ebola, and hepatitis B, as well as older vector-borne infections such as malaria, dengue, and yellow fever (Harper in press). The risk for infection works in both directions; humans have transmitted diseases to nonhuman primates, often with devastating consequences for already endangered animal populations. The problem is partly explained by the close evolutionary relationships between humans and other primates. We are apes, after all, and thus share many of the same vulnerabilities to certain kinds of microorganisms. But evolution only gives us part of the story. The rest involves the human hunting of nonhuman primates and encroachment onto their habitats.

The hunting of nonhuman primates for bushmeat poses a high risk for the transmission of new diseases, especially blood-borne pathogens transmitted during the butchering process (Wolfe et al. 2005). It is estimated that 4.5 million tons of bushmeat per year are extracted from the Congo Basin of West and Central Africa (see Figure 5.1). This meat is often consumed by the hunters and their families, or sold in local markets. Some bushmeat products also reach international markets, where the demand for exotic foods or medicinal ingredients can be quite high. Bushmeat hunting also occurs within the context of larger-scale political and economic processes. In Cameroon, for instance, hunting activities are tied to internationally supported logging activities, which have created roads that reach deep into animal habitats and populated their shrinking peripheries with migrant workers. Here, inequalities play a major role—for although bushmeat is consumed by all social classes, it is often the poorest and most socially marginalized who engage in the actual hunting and butchering. Thus we see how subsistence, settlement, and social organization influence high-risk practices for the entry of new infections into the human population.

Humans have been hunting wild animals for at least a hundred millennia, and our hominid ancestors did so for several million years before that. If we have been hunting for this long, then why would contemporary hunting pose any more danger for exposure to new infections? The answer may be that it is not any riskier for us now than it was for our prehistoric ancestors. However, the key difference lies in the interconnectedness of today's human populations. A Paleolithic hunter might contract an acute blood-borne pathogen while butchering his or her animal prey, but that pathogen could not spread far in an isolated group of twenty to thirty people. In contrast, today's bushmeat hunter has access to machines and markets that can spread the same pathogen around the world. Still, we should take care not to become overly alarmed, for it is unlikely that a single match will burn the entire world. Evolution usually occurs in smaller steps rather than larger leaps; so too with the evolution of pathogens from animal to human infection.

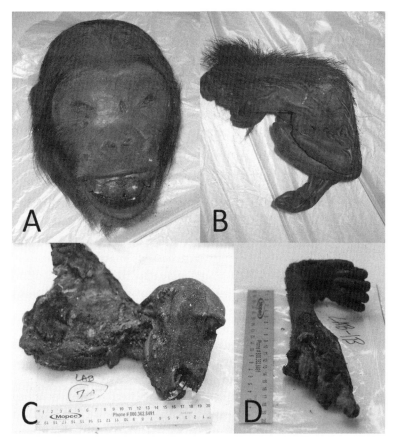

Figure 5.1. Nonhuman primate bushmeat specimens confiscated at US airports. Examples of smuggling simian bushmeat: a) skull; b) hand; c) skull and torso; d) arm. Ruler units are in centimeters. Smith, K.M. 2012. Zoonotic Viruses Associated with Illegally Imported Wildlife Products. *PLoS ONE* 7(1): e29505. doi:10.1371/journal.pone.0029505. Creative Commons Attribution 2.5.

Zoonotic pathogens must overcome at least three major challenges to mount a successful invasion and gain permanent entry in human host populations. First, they must somehow evolve animal-to-human transmissibility. Second, they must evolve human-to-human transmissibility. Finally, they must evolve the ability to be spread between human populations. These challenges correspond to three major stages: initial establishment, persistence, and spread (Anderson and May 1986). In the initial stage, infectious diseases can present some unique epidemiological features. One such feature is called "viral chatter," a term borrowed from intelligence agencies that monitor the "chatter" of electronic communications while searching for characteristic peaks in traffic regarding certain security-related topics (Wolfe 2011). Viral chatter occurs when a zoonotic pathogen first evolves the necessary characteristics for transmission from animal to human hosts, but not yet to the degree that the pathogen can be transmitted *between* human hosts. At this stage, the "chatter" consists of multiple, limited outbreaks among people in close contact with primary animal reservoirs. Viral chatter has been observed in the transmission of simian retroviruses to bushmeat hunters in Central Africa (Wolfe et al. 2004). It also explains phylogenetic evidence that HIV-1 and HIV-2 made at least ten incursions into the human population for a century before the arrival of the AIDS pandemic (Wolfe 2011).

Viral chatter reveals transitional moments in the co-evolution of pathogens and their future human hosts. For the pathogen species, evolution is strictly biological: a series of random mutations in which a very small percentage will confer reproductive advantages within certain environments. For instance, bacteria and viruses often enter and exit host tissues by the action of surface molecules (often referred to as antigens, if they have a role in the immune system). These antigens interact with their host cell like locks and keys. Sometimes the key does not fit the lock. Sometimes it does. And sometimes the key is specific to that particular new host, but cannot open further doors to infect another individual of the same species. For the human host, the evolution is primarily cultural such that individuals and groups engage in practices that create either bridges or barriers to possible infection. Bushmeat hunting creates bridges for animal to human infection, and more opportunities for pathogens to mutate until they develop a better key for the lock, thereby increasing the possibility of human-to-human transmission.

But as we consider these bridges for new pathogens, it is important that we not place too much weight on the role of unique or seemingly exotic cultural practices. In the early days of the AIDS pandemic, some irresponsible professionals implied that ritual voodun practices were the cause of a large cluster of Haitian cases (Farmer 1992). As it turned out, American sex tourists probably brought HIV to the island while seeking cheap sex from poor migrant workers in the capital city of Port-au-Prince (Farmer 1996). With a similar bias against cultural differences, a unique recipe was blamed for the inland spread of cholera during the 1992 epidemic in Peru. The marinated shellfish in Peruvian ceviche was thought to harbor the *Vibro* that had entered the city of Lima from the Pacific Ocean after being expelled from the bilge tanks of an offshore Chinese freighter. Consequently, sales of ceviche were temporarily banned. But not only did ceviche samples test free of cholera, the acidity of the local recipe was discovered to have a protective effect against infection (Tauxe et al. 1995). As with London in the mid-1800s, Lima's inadequate plumbing and drainage were primary conduits for the inland spread of cholera. Poverty and poor infrastructure contributed to the 1994 plague epidemic centered in the western Indian city of Surat, but local officials first attempted to deflect responsibility by propagating a rumor about international biowarfare experiments (Barrett 2006b).

Bushmeat hunting may indeed play an important role in the emergence of new pathogens, but we should also examine other, more common practices that have altered our relationships with potential animal hosts. Avian influenza ("bird flu") is an excellent example in this regard. We should first note that all influenza viruses are essentially avian influenzas insofar as they all infect bird hosts—from which they likely originated—while only some infect certain other animal species, and a few infect the human animal. The particular avian influenzas that have sparked so much concern are highly pathogenic among humans, with case fatality rates greater than 80 per cent for most outbreaks since 1997 (Barrett 2010). In addition, these viruses severely affect unusually large proportions of adolescents and young adults.[2] This age pattern is disturbingly similar to the 1918 influenza pandemic that killed 20–50 million people. Most seasonal influenzas exhibit a U-shaped pattern in which the very young and very old are most affected. Not so with the 1918 influenza, which exhibited more of a W-shaped curve with a peak of healthy young adults in the middle. So too with the highly pathogenic avian influenzas (HPAIs).

The good news is that these HPAIs are presently exhibiting little more than viral chatter in human populations. Of all the human HPAI cases detected since 1997, only a few might reasonably be attributed to human-to-human transmission (Wong and Yuen 2006). In addition, nearly all confirmed human cases of H5N1 avian influenza have thus far occurred as a result of bird-to-human transmission, with the highest risk for infection among poultry handlers (Dinh et al. 2006). The concern, however, is that one of these avian influenzas may someday evolve human-to-human transmissibility.

The bad news is that the influenza virus evolves rapidly, even by the standards of many other viruses. The genetic material (a genome) of influenza is made of RNA instead of DNA, a much more dynamic molecule that often reacts with itself as well as its surrounding molecules. Combine this with fast but sloppy replication systems, and we have a recipe for frequent mutations. These mutations are known as antigenic drift when they result in a change of surface molecules, particularly the hemaglutinin (H) and neuraminidase (N) molecules that allow the virus to get into and out of host cells. In addition to this, influenza viruses have multiple pieces of RNA (chromosomes) that can re-assort with those of different influenza viruses when more than one strain co-infects a single animal. These reshufflings are known as antigenic shift when they result in a change of surface molecules. It is because of these evolutionary dynamics, these drifts and shifts, that we must constantly develop new vaccines for new varieties of seasonal influenza.

Pigs have long been considered to be major living "mixing vessels" for the evolution of new human influenza varieties. This is because swine tissue surfaces (epithelia) contain receptors for both avian and human influenzas as well as their own (Ito et al. 1996). Swine have also been implicated in the H1N1 pandemic of 1918 as well as less severe pandemics of 1976 and 2009. Moreover, some researchers have blamed combined pig and duck farming practices in East Asia for the generation of new viruses. Yet although researchers have demonstrated these dynamics under laboratory conditions, the field evidence is less certain, and there are observations to suggest that antigenic shifts more often occur through seasonal mixing among migratory waterfowl (Morgan 2006).

More recently, biologists have examined the relative contributions of wild birds and domestic poultry to the spread of avian influenza (Kleinman et al. 2008). With high concentrations of virus particles (virions) in their intestinal tracts, wild bird species such as mallards

---

[2] There is evidence to suggest that an age-mediated hyper-inflammatory response ("cytokine storm") may explain unusually high mortality among young adults (Cheung et al. 2002), but this does not exclude other social factors, such as higher frequencies of exposure and psychological stress among working-age people in poorer populations.

and other waterfowl are known to disseminate influenza globally along migration routes (Olsen et al. 2006). Yet their migrations do not correlate well with human HPAI outbreaks, the latter of which were contained within China and South-east Asia until 2004 (Gauthier-Clerc et al. 2007). However, these same data show that many outbreaks closely correlate with transportation routes for the distribution of commercial poultry and poultry-based fertilizer products. Wild birds probably play important roles in mixing and long-range dissemination, but commercial poultry appear to be the primary reservoirs for human HPAIs.

This brings us back to Mike Davis' statement about the super-urbanization of the human species and its meat supplies (Davis 2006). The dilemma is exemplified by the world's commercial poultry industries (see Figure 5.2). At the time of the last major HPAI epidemic, there were about 12 billion chickens in East Asia, 70 per cent of which lived in high-density commercial poultry cages that provided 300 square centimeters of space per bird. These birds were consumed by human populations in urban densities up to 50 000 people per square kilometer. Thus, both humans and chickens have been squeezed into crowded settlements; both have been subjected to nutritional stressors, psychological stressors, and then buffered by an abundance of antimicrobial drugs. Except for the existence and use of these drugs, this situation is not qualitatively different from that of the First Epidemiological Transition. The scale is much larger, however, and with the condensation and convergence of human and avian habitats, opportunities for the emergence and spread of new infectious diseases are more extensive than those presented by any bird migration.

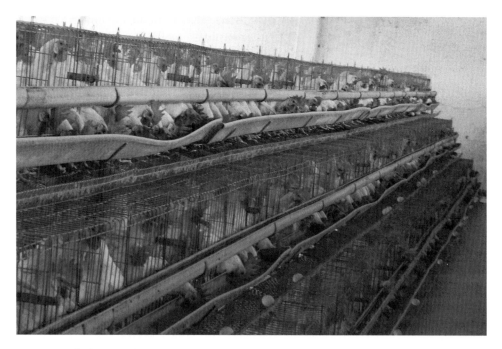

Figure 5.2. Chickens confined in battery cages in a mid-sized commercial poultry production facility in India. Photograph by Ron Barrett.

This brings us to even broader issues of human subsistence in the Third Transition. Out of more than 5000 plant species that have been used for human food, less than 150 species are represented in today's food markets. Moreover, less than twenty species comprise the majority of our food supply, and only three grains (wheat, rice, and corn) account for 60 per cent of the calories consumed by the human population (Armelagos 2010). This reduction of dietary diversity is also driven by indirect human consumption—that is, by the domesticated animals that eat the same plant foods in order to provide the world's meat supply. Worldwide, the human population consumes an average of 36.5 kilograms (about 80 pounds) of meat per person each year.

Of course, this average includes a substantial degree of variation. Whether by choice or by cost, many people consume little or no meat at all, but the average is driven up considerably by consumption in affluent societies. In the United States, for instance, the average annual meat consumption is comparable to the average body weight of an adult American male.[3] In 2009, 35 million cows, 150 million pigs, and 9 billion birds, mainly chickens and turkeys, were killed to provide meat for North American plates (Kolbert 2009). Such figures have produced staggering changes to world human and animal populations. Ten thousand years ago, humans and a small number of domesticated animals represented less than 0.1 per cent of the world's mammalian biomass. Today, we combine with our animal food supply to achieve a total of more than 90 per cent of the mammalian biomass (Vince 2011).

Given the scale and manner of our industrial meat production, we should not be surprised that it has become a major source of new human pathogens or pathogen varieties. In the United States alone, food-borne infections are responsible for 76 million illnesses, 325 000 hospitalizations, and 5000 deaths each year (Mead et al. 1999). Among these, 14 million cases and 1800 deaths can be attributed to a specific infectious pathogen. Novel food-borne infections include Creutzfeldt-Jakob disease (CJD), a fatal neurodegenerative condition caused by a protein-based agent known as a prion. A variant form of the disease (vCJD) has been experimentally linked to bovine spongiform encephalopathy (BSE), more popularly known as "mad cow disease," via consumption of contaminated beef (Gregor 2007). Commercially raised cattle are also known to carry E. coli 0157:H7. The toxin produced by this bacterium is harmless to cattle but potentially fatal to humans. Commercial meat has also been implicated in the emergence of *Campylobacter jejuni*, *Listeria monocytogenes*, and new disease agents from the Norovirus genus. We can also include a number of multi-drug-resistant pathogens, such as the bacterial *Enterococci*, as well as the transmission of drug-resistant genes to normal human flora, issues that we will address in the next chapter.

With increasing public awareness of these disease risks, many people are shifting away from mass-produced commercial foods. But these same foods are often the least expensive and most readily available. Many people cannot afford to eat otherwise, especially in urban areas. Also, the same inequalities that compel some people to butcher animals in rainforests also compel many others to butcher domesticated animals in large-scale production facilities. In

---

[3] About 88.6 kilograms, or 192 pounds.

both cases, steep hierarchies in the organization of human societies place certain groups of people at the riskiest junctures for the entry of new pathogens into our species. These inequalities continue to play a central role in the evolution of new pathogens: from those that dwell solely in nonhuman animals, to those that dwell across human populations.

5.2 Virulence and Vulnerability

A microbe does not become a pathogen until it makes us sick. This may seem an obvious point, but it becomes less so when we consider the number and diversity of microbial flora (microbiota) that reside upon and within the human body. Recall that each of our bodies is home to ten times as many bacterial cells as human cells. These include thousands of different bacterial species that dwell on our skin surfaces and within our guts (Ursell et al. 2012). The particular collection of species on the hand of one person has less than 20 per cent similarity to that on the hand of another person, even if the two are identical twins (Turnbaugh et al. 2010). Furthermore, the bacterial collection on your right hand share only about 14 per cent of the collection on your left hand (Fierer et al. 2008). Our bodies are menageries of microbiota, and these menageries are very different, even in similar and nearby places.

The vast majority of our microbiota is harmless, and many play important roles as "probiotics" in the maintenance of human health (Clemente et al. 2012). Skin and gut bacteria can provide immunological protection by competing against harmful invaders. One species, *B. fragilis*, helps regulate the immune system itself by producing a molecule that strikes a certain balance between pro-inflammatory and anti-inflammatory T cells. There are microbiota that can synthesize vitamins, such as vitamin B12, which we cannot produce on our own. There are some bacteria that help us digest complex carbohydrates so we can get more out of our food. Additionally, there is at least one bacteria, *Heliobacter pylori*, that helps regulate appetite when we have had enough. *H. pylori* also helps regulate stomach pH by providing negative feedback, much like a thermostat, against the overproduction of hydrochloric acid. But some people react differently to this feedback such that it leads to gastric ulcers and even stomach cancer. *H. pylori* is a good example of a microbe that is a probiotic in some contexts and a pathogen in others.

Even when they have no known benefit, there are a number of potential pathogens that do not usually make us sick. The most infamous of these is *M. tuberculosis*. It is estimated that 30 per cent of the human population has been exposed to this mycobacterium, yet 30 per cent of the world does not have tuberculosis. There are many factors to consider in the manifestation of TB, only one of which is the presence of the microbe. There are genetically determined factors that govern the physiological activities of both host and parasite. There are the circumstances of the infection itself, such as the initial amount or concentration (titer) of organisms, their path of entry into the human body, and the particular tissue and region colonized within the body. Crucially, there are host factors such as nutritional and immune states, possible co-infections, and other physical and psychological stressors.

Virulence is the degree to which a pathogen makes us sick. We can measure virulence according to mortality rates or the frequency and severity of pathological signs. Some researchers measure virulence according to the concentration of pathogens in the body. But this can be misleading because relatively small concentrations of certain pathogen varieties can make people very sick while larger concentrations of other varieties hardly make people sick at all—which is to say that their virulence is "attenuated." Whatever the method, it is important that we are clear about which criteria are being used to define the term. For the purposes of this book, we define virulence as the risk that a pathogen will cause the death of its infected host over a given period of time. Henceforth, the higher the virulence, the higher (or faster) the mortality.

For many years, biologists hypothesized that pathogens become more attenuated as they co-evolve with their hosts over time. The Attenuation Hypothesis was based on the reasoning that it would not be in the evolutionary interests of the microbe to kill its host too soon, or perhaps not at all, lest it be prematurely evicted from its place of residence (Ewald 1994). To adapt an old phrase, one should not bite too hard on the hand that feeds you, especially if you are a pathogen and your meal is the hand itself. Moreover, attenuation can increase opportunities for further spread as the same host remains contagious for a longer period of time. This explains why most heirloom and souvenir parasites of our Paleolithic ancestors usually caused chronic, non-lethal infections (Kliks 1990). With such small and geographically scattered populations, it was often many months before different foraging groups came into contact with one another. A pathogen could become extinct if it killed off one group before it had a chance to infect another. In the interim, it was far better for the parasite if the infected host was not only alive, but also well enough to walk long distances and interact with other potential hosts.

Attenuation was also a successful strategy for at least some infections of the First Transition. The smallpox virus was a good example of this—Variola having major and minor varieties. The minor variant was the more likely stowaway on the long journey from Old World to New World, and even more likely if it could hide undetected in an asymptomatic carrier. Jumping forward to the Third Transition, we see reverse examples of the same principle when a new human infection kills its hosts too quickly and too often. Since it was first detected in the late 1970s, the Ebola virus has only appeared in small and limited outbreaks. Primarily a blood-borne infection, Ebola shares the same major risk factors as HIV: contaminated needles and unprotected sex. But for HIV, the time from initial infection to serious illness is typically more than a decade, during which time the infected host carries high titers of the virus with no detectable symptoms. In contrast, Ebola infection rapidly develops into a severe and easily detectable illness that often progresses to death just as rapidly (Dowell et al. 1999). Consequently, the virus "flashes out" before it has a chance to sustain a long chain of infection and spread further in human populations.

Perhaps someday Ebola will evolve a strain that is less virulent to humans, but depending on circumstances, this might not be the virus's most successful evolutionary strategy. Attenuation or latency may work well for a pathogen, like smallpox, that makes its "living" on a single host species and cannot live anywhere else. However, a pathogen may have better options if it can move between multiple animal species or persist for long periods outside of any creature. Contrary to the Attenuation Hypothesis, one of these options may be to increase rather than decrease virulence, especially if increasing the symptoms somehow facilitates the further spread of the pathogen.

Bubonic plague is a good example of high virulence aiding the spread of infection, but here the victim is an insect. Plague is caused by the bacterium *Yersinia pestis*, a mostly zoonotic pathogen that typically circulates between biting insects and rodents in many parts of the world. It occasionally becomes "epizootic," infecting a small number of human individuals each year. In rare instances, it can cause larger outbreaks, which are usually self-limiting and usually associated with acute environmental disruptions (Barrett 2006b). Either way, the human victims are often cured with basic antibiotics. However, the insect victims are not so lucky. One of these victims is the rat flea (*Xenopsylla cheopis*), which typically contracts the disease by dining on the blood of its infected namesake. The bacteria then multiply in the gut of the flea until they form a large mass that completely obstructs the entry of any more food. Starving and ravenous, the flea bites even more animals while regurgitating bacteria, thereby spreading the disease to even more animal hosts.

We are not likely to shed tears over the death of a flea, but the same virulence strategy can also apply to human hosts. Paul Ewald, an evolutionary biologist, compared the mortality rates for human infections that were transmitted between humans via biting insects with those that were transmitted directly from human to human (Ewald 1983). He found a higher proportion of diseases with greater than 1 per cent mortality rates among the vector-borne infections than among the directly transmitted infections. Based on these data, Ewald concluded that evolution favored increasing virulence for pathogens that can survive in multiple hosts. But even though Ewald controlled for a number of variables, we cannot determine whether this study was based on a representative sample of diseases. There are contrary examples in which the directly transmitted variety of a disease is more virulent than its vector-borne variety. Again, plague is a good example; the directly transmitted, respiratory (i.e., pneumonic) form of plague is much more virulent than the vector-borne (bubonic) form of the disease, even though both are caused by the same pathogen.

As with the Attenuation Hypothesis, we should be careful not to over-generalize the Virulence Hypothesis. And as with most biological predictions, it is difficult to account for all the variables needed to predict future levels of pathogen virulence in human hosts. We already discussed some of the factors that can influence whether exposure to a pathogen leads to host infection. The same factors can apply to virulence insofar as they influence different stages in the transmission process, such as dispersion from the initial host, translocation to another susceptible host, and then colonization within that host. These factors include physiological characteristics of the pathogen, the genes for which can sometimes be transmitted between different microbial species via DNA or RNA segments known as plasmids, or by segments from a virus that infects a bacterium, processes that are generally known as horizontal gene transfer (HGT) (Gregor 2007). These genetic factors can be passed between pathogen strains or species, either directly, or via "third parties" such as the nonpathogenic flora of the human microbiota. We will see in the next chapter how these same mechanisms are implicated in the transmission of drug resistance.

Virulence can worsen disease symptoms, such as coughing, vomiting, and diarrhea, which can aid in the further dispersion of pathogens. Cholera is one such example. Most

Vibrio cholera do not cause disease in humans; they swim in oceans and other brackish waters, where they play an important ecological role in recycling carbon from the chitinous exoskeletons of plankton and other small creatures (Cottingham et al. 2003). The pathogenic varieties usually infect humans via the ingestion of unsanitary water and food, or by hand-to-mouth contact. Those that survive the stomach take up residence in the small intestine, where they latch on tightly to the epithelial lining with a hook-like appendage (Sack et al. 2004). They then secrete a toxin that causes the body to expel tremendous amounts of water, so much that a person can die of dehydration less than 36 hours after infection. Yet although this symptom is devastating to the host, it confers at least two advantages on the pathogen. The first is that it washes away competing bacteria that do not adhere so firmly to the gut lining. The second is that it disperses large quantities of *Vibrio* into the world—traveling through drainpipes, dwelling on living surfaces, or hitching a ride on other human caregivers.[4] Of course, such events are much less likely when people have access to clean water and adequate medical care.

The age-selective virulence of the 1918 influenza may have also aided the dispersion of the virus, which affected more people than any other known infection in history, killing at least 20 million people worldwide. Recall that the 1918 virus infected a larger proportion of young adults than most influenzas. In many societies, these were the most socially and geographically mobile age groups, especially during the First World War. They were thus likely to have the highest number of contacts for a given period of infectivity. There is evidence that this virus had a genetically coded virulence factor that causes a kind of hyper-immune reaction called a "cytokine storm" in the human respiratory lining, and that this reaction peaks in young adults (Cheung et al. 2002). But young adults were likely to be under additional stresses during a time of war, and the combatants themselves even more so as they lived and fought in open tranches for months at a time (Crosby 1989). There is also epidemiological evidence that co-infection with tuberculosis, which disproportionately affected young adult males, was a significant risk factor for the unusual age and sex ratios for influenza-related deaths at the time (Noymer and Garenne 2000).

Plague, cholera, and the 1918 influenza pandemic illustrate the complex dynamics of virulence and transmissibility. All three entail genetic adaptations of the pathogen. They also entail changes in host susceptibility, ecological interactions with other microorganisms, and the sociocultural factors that drive these changes and interactions. Yet even when we account for all these variables we are still unable to predict virulence with certainty. We can identify the high-risk conditions for plague, but we could not predict that the 1994 plague epidemic in western India would turn out to be relatively less virulent for its majority of pneumonic cases. We can also predict the high-risk conditions for cholera, but we could not know whether it would be the classic variety, the attenuated El Tor variety, or the deadly 0139 Bengal. And with influenza we never know, save to say that new varieties will emerge every year, and that, someday, we may have another large pandemic.

---

[4] Ewald refers to this as attendant-borne transmission, a useful concept, notwithstanding some shortcomings of his theory.

5.3 The Ancient Determinants of Future Pandemics

With all this focus on new and virulent infections, the question arises: when is the next pandemic and what will it be? The false optimism of the 1960s and 1970s is behind us now, and many health authorities point to the 1918 influenza pandemic as if it was a Krakatoa or Pompei—tragedies punctuating a recurring cycle of disasters in which it is only a matter of time until the next occurence. But even with this morbid certainty, we cannot predict the specifics: the pathogen, the time, the place, or the people. We did not know about SARS until it happened, and we had very little warning about the H1N1 outbreak of 2009. Both epidemics turned out to be self-limiting, but not because of the insightful actions of any population or government. In both cases, humanity dodged a bullet and learned few if any lessons from the experience.

The key lessons from this chapter are that microbial invasions do not occur all at once, and they do not occur in a vacuum. New pathogens evolve human transmissibility in stages, becoming "domesticated" much like the food animals and zoonotic pathogens of the Neolithic. This domestication process could be likened to that of cooking, in which living organisms are modified for entry into the human body, but with colonization rather than digestion as the evolutionary outcome. Here, the random mutations of pathogens result in modified surface proteins that allow access to, and exploitation of human tissues in competition with other organisms. These same mechanisms apply to the characteristics of virulence and latency, which can play major roles in the sustained transmission of these pathogens in human populations.

The good and bad news is that humans play major roles in these evolutionary processes. Whether for bushmeat or industrial meat, our subsistence practices continue to expose us to new strains and species of potential human pathogens. Population densities continue to drive the transmission of acute infections in super-urban communities, both human and animal. The inequalities in human societies create vulnerable populations for the entry and incubation of pathogens at the early stages of their invasions. These are the key points of intervention for the prevention of new and virulent infections, opportunities for action well before the chatter becomes the next major pandemic.

6

Inevitable Resistance

Except in a few situations, microorganisms are today as undisciplined a force of nature as they were centuries ago.

Mirage of health. *René Dubos (1959: 67)*

Microbes have been competing with each other for more than a billion years. Amid this competition, some evolved the ability to produce chemicals that inhibit or destroy their neighbors. Many of these chemicals are the basis for our antimicrobial drugs, and in some cases, these natural substances are the drugs themselves. Yet for as long as microbes have been competing with each other, they have also evolved ways to evade or resist these chemical assaults. Given this, we should not be surprised that pathogens have evolved defenses against our efforts to destroy them. But we have indeed been surprised, and even more so by how fast they have evolved these defenses.

Three years after penicillin was first introduced as the "magic bullet" and "wonder drug" against major bacterial infections, resistant strains of *Staphylococcus aureus* appeared in British and North American hospitals (Amyes 2001). In the next decade, *Streptococcus pneumoniae* followed suit, and the first strains of methicillin-resistant *Staph. aureus* (MRSA) appeared among hospitalized patients. Similarly, the first drug-resistant strains of *Mycobacterium tuberculosis*, and its cousin, *M. leprae*, appeared within a decade after antibiotics were introduced for TB and leprosy control. Today, many infections are multi-drug-resistant and many are endemic to communities around the world. Moreover, some diseases, like multi-drug- and extensively drug-resistant tuberculosis (MDR/XDR-TB), could become major pandemics if they are not soon brought under control (Kim et al. 2005).

Some have likened this problem to an arms race between humans and microbes, with the odds favoring the latter. Others have framed the problem in terms of host–pathogen evolution, a situation in which the rate of genetic adaptations among pathogens may exceed the rate of cultural adaptations among their hosts. Either way, it would seem that the unnatural history of drug resistance is nearly as long—or rather, as short—as the history of the medicines themselves. Resistance seems inevitable as we move toward a post-antibiotic era, a time when a dirty doorknob or simple scratch could result in an infection for which we would have no external defense (Garrett 1994).

This chapter examines the unnatural history of antibiotic resistance in light of the Third Epidemiological Transition. Here, we provide some anthropological approaches that are not

An Unnatural History of Emerging Infections. First Edition. Ron Barrett and George J. Armelagos.
© Ron Barrett and George J. Armelagos 2013. Published 2013 by Oxford University Press.

typically found in texts about the topic. One approach examines the antimicrobial role of some traditional medicines that pre-date modern biopharmaceuticals. Another examines how the biopharmaceuticals have influenced the way that people think about infectious diseases by overemphasizing the molecular characteristics of pathogens at the expense of attending to the social and environmental characteristics of human hosts. In so doing, policy-makers ignored key lessons from the decline of infectious diseases in the Second Transition.

We will consider how these lessons help to broaden our perspective on commonly cited issues in the emergence of drug resistance: the misuse of antibiotics in medicine and agriculture, and the problem of compromised immunity in vulnerable populations. We will again see how these issues are intimately tied to the ancient themes of human subsistence, settlement, and social organization. Finally, we will turn our gaze to the question of inevitable resistance—whether the current trends in the evolution of drug resistance can be reversed, or whether they will persist despite policy and behavioral changes. Either way, we must recognize that, in a global disease ecology, changes cannot be sustained anywhere unless they are applied everywhere.

6.1 Long Before Antibiotics . . .

Long before modern vaccines and antibiotics, societies around the world used a variety of traditional medicines for the treatment and prevention of infectious diseases (Plotkin 2005). Many of these medicines were effective, and some have since been adopted into the pharmacopeia of Western biomedicine. More than a thousand years before Edward Jenner gave his first vaccination, Indian Ayurvedic physicians and priests of the smallpox goddess, Shitala Ma, inoculated people by scratching the skin with scab preparations obtained from those infected with a milder strain of the virus, *Variola minor*. This method, later known as variolation, conferred partial immunity to the more deadly strain of the virus, *Variola major*.

The British royal family began variolating its members in the early 18th century, after which the practice was quickly adopted in Europe and North America. One well-publicized study at the time showed that people who had been variolated were ten times more likely to survive a *V. major* infection than those who were not (Klebs 1913). As a child, Jenner himself was inoculated using this ancient technique, which he later improved by substituting *V. minor* with *Vaccinia*, a strain closely related to cowpox (Hopkins 2002). Jenner received worldwide recognition for this improved method, which became known as vaccination. Yet even then, Jenner's "discovery" was based on earlier ethnomedical knowledge. English dairy farmers had long known about the protective effects of cowpox (Jenner 1798/2010).

Variolation was also practised throughout China for at least a dozen centuries. The inoculum was but one of many traditional Chinese medicines for boosting immunity and fighting fever-related diseases (Plotkin 2005). These traditional medicines included *Qinghao*, a tea prescribed for intermittent fevers. *Qinghao* was rediscovered in the 1960s by a joint team of Chinese pharmacologists and textual scholars who were seeking to develop new biomedicines from ancient remedies (Hsu 2006). One of *Qinghao's* main ingredients was an extract of

Artemisia annua—also known as "sweet wormwood" or "Sweet Annie"—a turquoise, fern-like herb with a camphor scent that is commonly found in temperate regions around the world. Further isolation and testing revealed that a particular compound within the wormwood, artemisinin, is highly effective for treating malaria, schistosomiasis, and other parasitic infections. Presently, the World Health Organization recommends artemisinin, in combination with other drugs, as a first-line therapy for Falciparum malaria—the form of the disease associated with the highest number of deaths worldwide (World Health Organization 2010a).

In addition to the use of antimicrobial herbs, at least some ancient societies ingested what we would consider to be a proper antibiotic today. In the late 1970s, Debra Martin was conducting her doctoral research in biological anthropology, examining bone remodeling to further our understanding of the health of Sudanese Nubians who lived along the Nile River between 350–550 CE. At one point, she needed a standard light microscope to check her measurements on some very thin sections of bone. None was available, so she resorted to an ultraviolet microscope, and was surprised to see a yellow-green glow at a particular wavelength that indicated tetracycline molecules bound to the calcium within the tissue. Further chemical analysis revealed that this was indeed the case (Bassett et al. 1980). It was like unwrapping a mummy, only to find the corpse wearing earphones and a pair of sunglasses.

There is, however, a plausible explanation for this fantastic discovery. Like most first-generation antibiotics, tetracycline is a naturally occurring substance excreted by soil microbes, probably as an adaptive mechanism for gaining advantage over other competing species. This mechanism is called antibiosis, the namesake of modern antibiotics. Even so, Martin's discovery was met with some disbelief. Because of its natural origins, the tetracycline in the Nubian skeletons could have resulted from process known as taphonomic infiltration: postmortem contamination by invading microorganisms that occurred as the bodies decomposed, or during the centuries while they were buried in the ground (Piepenbrink et al. 1983).

However, infiltration was unlikely in the case of these Nubian bodies. The analysis of collagen and osteons indicates little contamination of these remains; natural mummification resisted invading organisms. Furthermore, closer examination revealed patterns of deposition that are consistent with long-term tetracycline ingestion by living people (Nelson, et al. 2010). These patterns clearly indicate long-term tetracycline consumption during the formative stages of bone development during the early years of life. Similar evidence has been found in neighboring societies: a 2000-year-old Jordanian population, and a group of Egyptians living under Roman occupation between 400 and 500 CE (Armelagos et al. 2001).

Although we know these societies consumed tetracycline, we can only hypothesize their means or motives for doing so. Bread and beer are plausible vehicles. Both were staple foods, the beer having been brewed for nutrition more than intoxication. Some ancient Egyptian and Nubian recipes include steps that could easily lead to the molding of grains similar to the blue, penicillin-like streaks found on certain cheeses. Two undergraduates at Emory University demonstrated how these recipes could produce tetracyclines by experimentally adding *Streptomycetes* organisms at various stages of the cooking process (Armelagos et al. 2001). As to motives, some Egyptian texts prescribe beer as a treatment for a variety of ills such as gum disease, vaginitis, and wound infections. But while these data are suggestive, further research is needed to determine if any of these groups deliberately consumed tetracy-cline compounds for health purposes.

We should not be surprised by these ancient discoveries. Throughout the world's ecosys-tems, biologists have identified hundreds of plant and animal substances with antimicrobial activities (Rios and Recio 2005). We can reasonably predict that people who have lived in these environments would have made similar discoveries through trial and error over many generations. Indeed, pharmaceutical companies often bank on this prediction. Rather than conduct undirected surveys of the world's flora and fauna, which would be impractical and expensive, these companies send people to far corners of the globe to gather ingredients from traditional medicines. The ingredients are then brought back to the laboratory, where their constituent compounds are extracted, isolated, and tested for biomedical efficacy. These activities are collectively known as pharmacognosy, or by the more popular terms, "bio-prospecting" and "medicine hunting."

Pharmacognosy, the search for natural or traditional medicines, has proven to be quite successful. Of the 210 small molecule drugs in the World Health Organization's List of Essential Medicines, 139 of these substances have been derived or modified from natural sources (Jones et al. 2006). Most of these substances have been used as ingredients for traditional medi-cines. That said, pharmacognosy has at least two significant shortcomings. The first concerns intellectual property rights. All too often, traditional healers and their communities do not receive sufficient credit or economic benefit from these discoveries, if any at all (Ellen 1995). The second shortcoming of pharmacognosy is its exclusive focus on finding individual (pat-entable) molecules rather than considering the broader contexts in which traditional medi-cines are used (Etkin 1996). These contexts include the interactions of therapeutic substances with other elements of the healing process, not just the pharmacological ones, and the place of these therapies in particular belief systems and social relationships. Such broader investi-gations are typically performed by ethnopharmacologists, specially trained ethnographers who attempt to bridge our cultural and biological understandings of traditional healing. Unlike the pharmacognocist, the ethnopharmacologist typically operates outside the finan-cial interests of the pharmaceutical industry.

It is difficult to summarize the findings of ethnopharmacology without running the risk of over-generalization. That said, we can identify a few common themes in these studies of tra-ditional healing systems, even if the themes are by no means universal. Some follow the pre-dictions above: that societies who develop biologically effective medicines have typically done so after observing the effects of different substances on the human body over the course of many generations. Another is that the accumulated wisdom of these observations need not rely on biomedical beliefs about why these medicines work. Indeed, the same can be said for biomedicine itself. In most industrialized countries, years of research and bureaucratic hur-dles are required to approve a biomedicine for official use. But all these efforts are focused on how the drug works, not why it works the way it does. Browse any biomedical drug reference, and you will find approved medications for which the mechanisms of action are not yet known. In these cases, biomedicine relies on empirical observations independent of its own theories. The empiricism may be more systematic, but the overall approach is essentially the same as many other non-biomedical healing traditions.

Lastly, traditional medicines are frequently based on extensive ecological knowledge. In Chapter 1, we saw how the subsistence practices of non-literate foraging societies require detailed knowledge of flora and fauna in order to meet people's nutritional needs in diverse and changing environments. The same could be said for the environmental knowledge required to meet people's therapeutic needs. Brent Berlin's comprehensive study of traditional taxonomies reflects this kind of ecological knowledge, with foraging societies describing a greater number and variety of taxa than agricultural societies in the same local environments (Berlin 1992). Many of these taxa are, in turn, associated with health and disease categories of belief systems that emphasize people's relationships to one another and the species around them—indigenous theories of human ecology.

Human ecology is also a common theme of major textual healing traditions (Hsu and Barrett 2009). Indian Ayurvedic medicine considers human health characteristics based on factors such as seasonal climates, personal habits, and interpersonal relationships, as well as the different balances of humor-like *doshas* that govern all living creatures in the middle world. Traditional Chinese medicine accounts for similar health factors in the context of five winds, dynamic balances of *yin* and *yang*, and flows of *qi* energy that permeate the natural and supernatural alike. Tracing the origins of their practice to Classical Greece, the Islamic healers of *Unaani Tib* emphasize the importance of human constitutions based on the particular social and physical environments in which people were raised, principles reflected in the writings of Galen and Hippocrates.

Hippocrates, the putative father of Western biomedicine, strongly emphasized the broader ecologies of human health. Biomedicine, however, has since moved toward a more focused approach, devoting much of its attention to individual causes, for individual diseases, of individual humans—all removed from their environmental contexts. This was not always the case.

6.2 From Soil and Seed to Magic Bullets

Writing in the last years of the 19th century, Timothy McGillicuddy, a New York obstetrician, drew on agricultural metaphors to describe the most likely conditions for a TB infection. In deference to Germ Theory, he acknowledged the recently discovered microbacterium to be the "seed" of the disease, stating that *M. tuberculosis* had been "defined and described until there is no more doubt as to its nature and characteristics than there is about a grain of wheat" (Mcgillicuddy 1898: 1396). But as with the wheat grain, this microorganism "does not always sprout where it falls; if the tubercle bacillus attacked everyone exposed to its influence, the [human] race would have been exterminated ere this. Not only seed but soil is essential to the crop" (McGillicuddy 1898: 1396).

McGillicuddy's ideas were widely shared among his peers. By the time of his writing, seed and soil were popular metaphors among increasing numbers of European and North American physicians who had recently converted from miasma theory to contagionism, but still continued to recognize the importance of pre-existing health conditions and surrounding environments for the development of infectious disease (Barnes 1995). As we saw in Chapter 3, contagionists and anti-contagionists had been waging a hard-fought battle since the mid-19th century—a conflict fueled by social and economic considerations as much as the ambiguity of scientific evidence (Ackerknecht 1948/2009). By the 1880s, Germ Theory was largely accepted by the biomedical community. But despite growing academic emphasis on the microscopic seeds of infection, the clinical practice of biomedicine was still firmly rooted in the soil of sanitary reform.

We know that Germ Theory does not exclude sanitary practice. Indeed, the discovery of pathogens further supported the virtue of clean environments for preventing disease transmission. As such, the dual recognition of seed and soil could have informed a new holistic approach to infection, one that considered the interactions between microscopic and macroscopic worlds. But these metaphors did not signal a holistic perspective so much as a disjuncture between theory and practice. Soil and seed informed different kinds of medical activities: one was academic, the other was clinical.

On the academic side, microbiologists were discovering new pathogens at every turn, but on the clinical side, Germ Theory offered little new for the practice of medicine until well into the 20th century. Robert Koch discovered *M. tuberculosis* sixteen years before Dr McGillicuddy wrote about the soil and seed of consumption, but it would be another forty years before the development of effective biomedicines for this disease. In the absence of such developments, McGillicuddy believed that the best therapy was to cleanse the body of contaminants and provide exercise, rest, and good nutrition. He felt the latter was especially important, stating an old maxim: "If you take care of the stomach, the lungs will take care of themselves" (1899: 1397). McKeown would have approved of these measures, as they were largely responsible for the decline of infectious diseases from the beginning of the Second Epidemiological Transition to the end of the Second World War (1974).

In the early 20th century, biomedical attention began shifting from the interactions of seed and soil, to the characteristics of the seeds alone as a new medicines were being developed that were selectively toxic to pathogens. Guided by Koch's success in identifying *M. tuberculosis*, Paul Ehrlich focused on selective staining techniques for visualizing particular microorganisms. Ehrlich hypothesized that the unique characteristics of bacterial walls allowed them to absorb, or adhere to, certain stains and dyes while the cells of surrounding tissues could not. Ehrlich reasoned that some of these stains and dyes might also be selectively toxic to bacteria, thereby killing pathogens while leaving the host unharmed. Inspired by the self-guided projectiles of Norse mythology, Ehrlich called these selective toxins "magic bullets" (Winau et al. 2004).

The magic bullet approach proved contagious with the early successes of Ehrlich and his colleagues (Amyes 2001). Ehrlich developed an arsenic-based compound known as Salvarsan (also known as arsphenamine or Compound 606) which had more success against syphilis and African trypanosomiasis than any previous treatment. Ehrlich's former assistant, Julius Morgenroth, discovered a quinine-derived dye, known as Optochin, that not only stained *Streptococcus pneumoniae* but also inhibited its growth. Gerhard Domagk had even better success against *S. pneumonia* with a red dye derivative called Prontonsil. That said, these early drugs had significant side effects; many people could not tolerate Salvarsan, and Optochin was never used medicinally due to its risk for blindness. Prontosil was a notable exception, however, proving very effective against strep infections with few side effects, and famously so when Franklin Roosevelt's son was stricken with a bad case of tonsilitis. Protonsil was the first of an entire class of sulfa drugs that are still in use today.

Penicillin gave the magic bullet concept its biggest boost. The story of Alexander Fleming's accidental discovery is the stuff of textbook legend, but it should also be noted that Fleming was well trained to look for the accident, having earlier studied the bacterial growth-inhibiting effects of lysozyme in human tears. Moreover, the significance of Fleming's discovery went unrecognized for more than a decade until a team of chemists found a way to purify the substance in a stable and medically useful form (Goldsworthy and McFarlane 2002). Following the Second World War, penicillin became widely distributed among the public, for whom it was touted as the "wonder drug" that could not only kill infections, but also prevent baldness and tooth decay. There was even a penicillin lipstick for those concerned about "hygienic kissing" (Brown 2004).

Quackery aside, penicillin was one the greatest biomedical contributions of the 20th century. The drug effectively killed many gram-positive organisms, including the ubiquitous staph and strep infections. It still continues to be the preferred treatment for primary syphilis. All told, penicillin is thus far responsible for saving more than a 100 million lives (Amyes 2001). In addition, the core molecule has served as the basis for the development of many subsequent drugs. Perhaps more importantly, penicillin opened the door to an entirely new area of medical inquiry, one that sought new medicines in the natural defenses of microorganisms.

No drug is free from the risk of side effects. In the case of penicillin, this risk has been epistemological as well as physiological. The success of penicillin enshrined the magic bullet concept in the teaching and practice of biomedicine, displacing other more holistic approaches that included both seed and soil. Since then, the majority of medical research funding (public and private) has been devoted to the molecular characteristics of pathogens rather than the states of human hosts and their surrounding environments. Moreover, the language used to think about these problems has become increasingly militaristic, such that medicines are seen as weapons for destroying enemy diseases. As a result, our theories of disease have been reduced to simple problems with single causes and convenient solutions—the latter being heavily marketed by the pharmaceutical industry.

The immanent microbiologist, Rene Dubos, referred to this reductive approach as the "Doctrine of Singular Etiology." He believed this doctrine was largely responsible for the naïve optimism that biomedical science would eventually cure all human ills, infectious diseases among them (Dubos 1959). In contrast to this approach, Dubos promoted an ecological view of humans and microbes as participants in a complex web of interactions that can sometimes benefit certain species at the expense of others. Dubos applied this ecological view in the laboratory, developing a method for isolating and identifying antibiotic-producing organisms amid the many microbial species living in soil and other natural sources. This method was used in the discovery of nearly every core antibiotic molecule since erythromycin (Amyes 2001). It is ironic that people would place so much faith in the medicinal fruit of Dubos' ideas while ignoring the ideas themselves.

6.3 Antibiotics and Human Use

Resistance may be as old as life itself, but humanity is accelerating the process. We can see this acceleration in the laboratory when bacteria are streaked on an agar plate (also known as a petri dish) that has been covered with an antibiotic. Depending on the drug and the organism, the antibiotic can kill or inhibit nearly all the bacteria on the plate. Now let us suppose that one in a billion of these bacteria develops a mutation that confers resistance to the antibiotic. This may seem like a very rare mutation, but it would mean the survival of a dozen mutants if 12 billion bacteria were streaked on the plate. Furthermore, these dozen mutants could then multiply exponentially until they produced a dozen plainly visible spots, each representing billions more bacteria, all within a single day.

This experiment clearly demonstrates natural selection in action. Here, a variant trait in a species becomes adaptive insofar as it confers a reproductive advantage in a selective environment. But it also demonstrates a form of artificial selection insofar as the conditions have been deliberately manipulated to accelerate the process. The bacteria are grown in the plate with little or no competition from other microbial species, which might otherwise have overgrown the study species under the same conditions. Furthermore, either the antibiotic or its concentration has to be less than 100 per cent effective. Otherwise, it would not have provided an opportunity for the production of new mutants in the first place.

We perform artificial selection every time we use an antibiotic and do so even more when we misuse an antibiotic. Misuse usually falls into one of two categories: underuse and overuse. Underuse is relatively easy to identify, even if its solutions are difficult. It occurs much like the previous experiment, when people use antibiotics that are less than completely effective against the particular species or strain that is infecting them, or more commonly, when they take sporadic doses or terminate therapy prematurely. Unlike the previous experiment, however, the evolution of resistance does not usually happen in a single stage. More often, it occurs in a series of stepwise changes from sensitivity to resistance. Here, the underuse of antibiotics allows for the survival of some organisms that would otherwise be killed. Among the survivors, the mutants with partial resistance (also known as "incomplete sensitivity") are present in larger numbers than those that are not. A larger dose of the antibiotic is needed to kill these partly resistant organisms—what biologists refer to as the minimum inhibitory concentration (or MIC) of the drug (see Figure 6.1). The MIC increases with each of these iterations until it reaches a level that is toxic to the human host. It is at this stage that the organism is considered resistant to the antibiotic.

The potential solutions to this problem are often more challenging than they first appear. The solutions to underuse may be a matter of educating health providers and their patients, but edu-

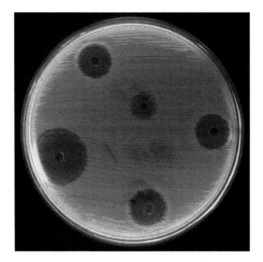

Figure 6.1. A drug-sensitivity test, with five antibiotic substances placed on an agar plate that has been covered with *Staphylococcus aureus* bacteria. The clear circles around the drugs indicate areas of inhibition against the bacteria. The concentration of the drug diminishes as it diffuses from the center, until reaches the minimum inhibitory concentration (MIC) where it can no longer prevent bacterial growth. More sensitive bacteria leave wider rings, while more resistant bacteria would leave no clear rings at all. Photograph by Don Stallons. U.S. Centers for Disease Control and Prevention.

cation is not simply about pouring knowledge into an empty vessel. For education to be effective, it must be meaningful and relevant to people's beliefs and practices, many of which may be more accurate or more effective than those of biomedicine. Patients may have histories of distrust or miscommunication with their providers, requiring a gradual rebuilding of these relationships over time. Even when these other factors are addressed, however, poor access to medical resources often results in underuse when the specific pathogen is not identified and people lack the information or proper medicine for treating the infection. Limited access to proper medicines can occur due to poor and unregulated manufacturing practices of small pharmaceutical companies; it can also occur due to poor distribution practices of large pharmaceutical corporations—in fact, these practices are often linked to one another. Any and all these factors can favor the odds of pathogen survival and continued evolution of antibiotic resistance.

The same factors apply to the overuse of antibiotics, but with the added challenge that the problem can be much harder to identify and define. Even when antibiotics are properly administered, the massive scale of their adoption by human societies around the world could be arguably defined as overuse. In 1954, the United States alone produced about a half million pounds of antibiotics; by 2000, this figure increased to 50 million pounds (Levy 2002). It is estimated that antibiotics comprise 70 per cent of all biopharmaceuticals consumed worldwide, adding up to US$26.5 billion in global sales in 2008, with an expected increase of 7 per cent over the next ten years (Gootz 2010). It is reasonable to predict that these quantities, even when appropriately prescribed, could inevitably lead to antibiotic resistant strains.

The problem is reflected in Figure 6.2, where we can see the emergence of antibiotic strains only a few years after the discovery and adoption of the medicines. Many of the earlier examples in this table were not so widely available that they could be easily misused, but again, the sheer quantity of the use of these drugs was bound to cause resistance. This would not be so troubling if the technical achievements of our species were outpacing the evolution of our pathogens. Unfortunately, this has not been the case; all major antibiotic classes are associated with at least one microbial resistance mechanism. Even more troubling, the last time we discovered a new core antibiotic molecule was in 1961—more than fifty years ago. Clearly, the microbial adaptations are outpacing the human adaptations (see Figure 6.3). In light of this, should we consider our present rate of antibiotic consumption to be overuse? Should we not slow things down?

Global health recommendations for decreasing antibiotic consumption include curtailing use for prophylaxis and for typically self-resolving infections such as non-febrile diarrhea or pediatric ear infections (World Health Organization 2007). Prophylactic use may be the easiest to forgo, as patients are not yet faced with difficult symptoms. But it may be more difficult to avoid antibiotics for minor infections, especially for the world's impoverished majority who lack both the time and the money to give up days of productive work when quick relief can be found with a few generic pills costing less than half a day's wages. People in developing countries often have poor access to professional medical providers, but they can often purchase cheap antibiotics without a prescription.

Another major form of overuse is the consumption of antibiotics that have no efficacy against the infection, such as when an antibiotic for one class of bacteria is used for another,

Antibiotic deployment

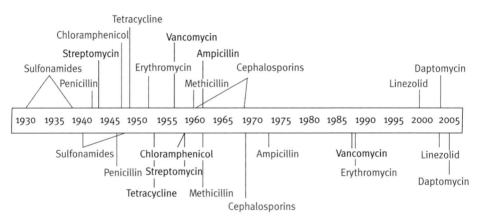

Antibiotic resistance observed

Figure 6.2. Time line of the development of twelve major antibiotics and the emergence of resistance to those same drugs. Clatworthy, Ann, Emily Pierson, and Debra T Hung 2007. *Nature Chemical Biology* 3, 541–548. Published online: 20 August 2007<doi:10.1038/nchembio.2007.24> Reproduced with permission from Nature Publishing Group.

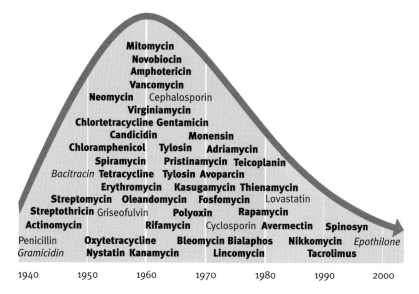

Figure 6.3. Time line illustrating the rate of antibiotic development from 1940–2000. The rate of antibiotic development has tapered in recent decades while that of antibiotic resistance has increased. Shetty, Priya 2008. *Antibiotic Resistance*. SciDevNet. Last accessed 12/02/2012.

or quite commonly, when it is used for a virus for which antibiotics have no effect whatsoever. These behaviors are certainly wasteful and possibly detrimental to a patient who might otherwise find a better treatment. Yet in terms of resistance, they might seem relatively harmless insofar as they could do no worse for an already resistant pathogen. Not so, however, when we recall the phenomenon of horizontal gene transfer (HGT) from the previous chapter.

In the same ways that many bacteria can transfer genes for virulence, they can also transfer genes for antibiotic resistance between one another. As with virulence genes, resistance genes can be encoded into plasmids, transposable sequences, and even viruses that infect bacteria. Now consider that antibiotics create, not only a selective environment for pathogens, but also for many species of commensal bacteria in our bodies. Some of these commensal species evolve antibiotic resistant genes, which they can then transfer to potential pathogens. Others pass these genes on, having acquired them from previous infections, or from other resistant microflora that had been growing in antibiotic-laden foods—a topic which we will address shortly. In the interim, it is important to note that the genes for pathogen resistance can be as contagious as the pathogens themselves, and the spread of these genes is strongly mediated by the ways we use and misuse antibiotics.

6.4 Antibiotics and Agricultural Use

Stuart Levy teaches antibiotic resistance with a tomato. A physician and leading researcher on the topic, Levy has his medical students conduct an experiment in which they slice a tomato with a sterile knife, briefly touch it to an agar plate covered with nutrients, and then incubate the plate overnight at body temperature. By the next morning, the plate is speckled with visible colonies of bacteria from the tomato, 10 per cent of which are resistant to one or more antibiotics; this, without the selective presence of any antibiotics in the first place (Levy 2002). In a field study of Boston food markets, Levy and his colleagues found 10 000 to 100 000 antibiotic resistant bacteria for each gram of vegetable they sampled. While none of these bacteria were harmful, 10–20 per cent were capable of colonizing human intestines, where they could transfer resistance genes to other potentially pathogenic species.

How did these bacteria become resistant? It might have been because of antibiotics used in growing the plants. Commercial food growers in the United States use 100 000 pounds of antibiotics a year for fruit trees alone, the equivalent of 45 million daily human doses. Even larger quantities are used for domesticated animals. About 15–17 million pounds of antibiotics are administered to thirty times more animals than humans in the United States each year. Moreover, these antibiotics are mostly used as growth factors in sub-therapeutic doses, often at 1–10 per cent of the amount needed to cure most infections. Nor is the United States alone in these practices. Multiply these doses for nearly all the world's large-scale animal growers, and we have massive selection for antibiotic resistance.

The use of antibiotics as an animal growth factor was discovered by accident in the 1950s. Chickens that were fed a vitamin B12 supplement put on more weight at faster rates than those that were not. However, it turned out that the supplement was contaminated with tetracycline, which was responsible for the accelerated growth. The most accepted explanation for this phenomenon is that the antibiotic suppresses large quantities of commensal bacteria that help digest plant cellulose in exchange for their share of the meal. Commercial feed does not require such digestion, so the bacteria become a liability. Suppress these bacteria, and the animals obtain more energy per meal, thereby resulting in faster growth (Amyes 2001).

Commercial agriculture is highly competitive, and farmers operate on narrow profit margins. A few days' difference in growth rates can spell success or ruin for a farmer or commodities trader. Consequently, antibiotic growth factors have become an essential ingredient in commercial agriculture (Figure 6.4). Following major studies about the impact of these practices on the emergence of drug-resistant bacteria, many countries, including those of the European Union, have passed regulations against using antibiotics as growth factors if they are commonly prescribed for human patients (Amyes 2001). The United States, however, has not yet passed such regulations. It is therefore not surprising that by the late 1980s, the rate of tetracycline resistance in the E. coli of food producing animals in the US was 96 per cent, and rate for ampicillin resistance was 77 per cent. Ampicillin and its sister compounds are some of the most widely prescribed antibiotics in the world.

Even the agricultural use of nonhuman antibiotics can pose significant risks. Many of these molecules resemble their human counterparts, and many resistance mechanisms apply to similar molecules. For example, strains of vancomycin-resistant *Enteroccocus faecium* were found in Danish farm animals that had been taking avoparcin (Bager et al. 2000). Although avaparcin is a nonhuman antibiotic growth factor, the molecule is very similar to

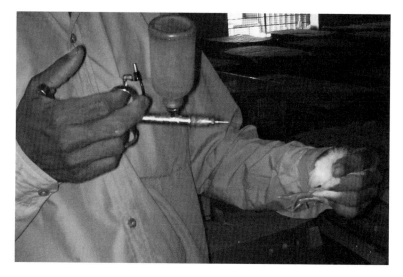

Figure 6.4. The use of antibiotics as growth factors is commonly practised in commercial animal-food production facilities around the world. Here, we see a worker administering antibiotics to baby chick in a commercial poultry facility in India. Photograph by Ron Barrett.

that of vancomycin. This finding is particularly troubling because vancomycin is often reserved as an antibiotic of last resort for infections that might otherwise be incurable, such as MRSA. Similarly, the use of ciprofloxin-like growth factors has resulted in cipro-resistant *Camphylobacter* strains in commercial poultry (Luangtongkum et al. 2009). Ciprofloxin and its related compounds are among the leading broad-spectrum antibiotics for serious gastrointestinal infections, lower respiratory infections, urinary tract infections, and gonorrhea.

In Chapter 5, we examined the super-urbanization of food animals and the consequences it poses for the amplification and spread of new and virulent infections. The same principle applies to the amplification and spread of antibiotic resistance. At present, about 30 per cent of all large-scale commercial poultry are infected with salmonella. Most of these strains have little or no effect on the animals. Nevertheless, some of these strains are resistant to as many as five different antibiotics (Amyes 2001). These strains can be passed to humans through the consumption of meat and eggs, causing severe and sometimes life-threatening infections.

Returning to the tomato, we should note that even the staunchest organic vegan is at risk for the drug-resistant consequences of commercial animal production. The average commercially raised dairy cow produces more than a hundred times the feces of the average human. As such, they are potential "factor[ies] for the production and dispersion of antibiotic resistant bacteria" (Marshall and Levy 2011: 719). Multiply these cows by a billion and you have 60 per cent of the world's total biomass of manure from domesticated animals. Include the rest, and that total comes to about 13 billion tons of manure per year— about two thousand times the mass of the Great Pyramid at Giza. Much of this waste becomes fertilizer, leaching into groundwater, channeling through irrigation canals, and contaminating drinking supplies in affluent as well as poor countries around the world.

Consequently, resistance is unavoidable. Ten thousand years ago, the domestication of animals brought us acute infectious diseases. Today, the medication of these same animals has brought us drug resistance, which is as contagious as the diseases themselves.

6.5 Antibiotics and Vulnerability

There is no such thing as a drug-resistant "superbug." On the contrary, drug-resistant bacteria are usually less hearty than non-resistant strains of the same species. This is because drug-resistance traits are energetically expensive, and usually more so in the case of multi-drug resistance. For instance, bacterial membranes may become less permeable, thereby restricting the entry of certain antibiotics, but that decreased permeability often restricts the entry of nutrients as well. Bacterial ribosomes that are slightly distorted may make them "invisible" to certain antibiotics, but these distortions also make them less efficient in helping to synthesize proteins. Certain bacterial enzymes may destroy antibiotic molecules, but their production also diverts energy and resources away from self-maintenance and reproduction. Such traits are a liability in the absence of antibiotics. Far from conferring super-powers, resistance is a drag for bacteria under normal conditions.

The cost of resistance explains three important epidemiological observations. The first is that humans may harbor multi-drug-resistant pathogens without knowing it. One study found that patients developed multi-drug-resistant *Salmonella* infections after taking antibiotics for other kinds of infections (Levy 2002). It turned out that these patients had already been carrying the *Salmonella* in their intestines, possibly for years. But these *Salmonella* were kept in check by the more competitive microbiota around them, subsisting in numbers too low to cause infection. After taking the antibiotics, the competition was suppressed and the *Salmonella* populations surged.

The second observation pertains to our earlier discussion about the underuse of antibiotics and the gradual evolution of drug resistance. Evolution often occurs through incremental changes, but these increments are likely to be smaller if the overall change is expensive. The same can be said for other biological traits, such as human-to-human transmissibility. If the changes needed to invade a human population are expensive, then the invasion may occur in smaller steps; the more cost, the more chatter. Yet by the same token, these changes are more likely to occur with bigger leaps and at faster rates if they are made cheaper by surrounding conditions. The best way to do this is by increasing the vulnerability of human hosts.

This brings us to the third observation: antibiotic-resistant infections usually appear first, and spread further and faster in the most vulnerable human populations. We see this in the emergence and spread of MDR-TB and XDR-TB. Ordinary tuberculosis is already a major disease of poverty; at present, 98 per cent of all TB deaths occur in developing countries (Kim et al. 2005). TB is also a major AIDS-defining illness, responsible for one-third of all deaths among HIV-infected people worldwide. TB has long been curable with a combination of three antimicrobial drugs. But just as the under-treatment of one person can lead to drug resistance, so too can the under-treatment of the world, only on a much larger scale. Humanity has been missing the window of opportunity for worldwide TB treatment, resulting in the spread of drug-resistant TB in these same impoverished and co-infected populations, comprising an estimated 440 000 cases globally in 2008, and more than 10 per cent of all TB cases in five countries (World Health Organization 2010b). The cost of treatment is twenty to thirty times higher for resistant than non-resistant infections. But the cost of non-treatment will be even higher if these resistant infections continue to spread.

Alexander Fleming warned that the misuse of penicillin could result in penicillin-resistant strains of *Staphylococcus aureus*. Within a year, the first resistant strains of *Staph. aureus* appeared in a British hospital ward (Amyes 2001). Within the next decade, strains began to appear that were resistant to methicillin, the next line of penicillin compounds. But MRSA was a rare infection for many years thereafter, mainly appearing among cancer patients undergoing chemotherapy. Then, in the 1980s, it began appearing among AIDS patients and elderly residents of nursing homes. Now MRSA is endemic to long-term care facilities and strains resistant to third-line penicillins are a common threat in hospitals, even in the world's most affluent societies. However, MRSA spreads more frequently in vulnerable populations, whether they are pneumonia patients that expel the bacterium via the cloud effect, or over-worked care-givers who are too tired and frustrated to wash their hands between patients. Resistance comes cheap under these conditions.

6.6 The Persistence of Resistance

Is resistance inevitable? One way to answer this question is to observe the continued evolution of drug-resistant bacteria in the laboratory after the removal of antibiotics. Given the biological cost of many resistant mechanisms, we would expect these mutations to revert back to their original drug-sensitive forms in the absence of selection pressure. Unfortunately, however, many bacterial resistance mechanisms have been much slower to disappear under these conditions than the rates at which they arose in the first place. Microbiologists refer to this phenomenon as the persistence of resistance.

Several mechanisms have been proposed to explain the persistence phenomenon. The first is that some resistance mechanisms may not be as costly as originally expected; this has turned out to be the case for a ribosomal mutation in *Staph. aureus* that confers resistance to seven antibiotics but without any growth reduction in an antibiotic-free environment (LaMarre et al. 2011). While these no-cost mutations are exceptions to the rule, they are more likely to occur when the resistance mechanism confers some other advantage under special circumstances, as is the case for certain strains of streptomycin-resistant Salmonella that grow more slowly but survive longer in low-protein environments (Andersson and Hughes 2011).

A second mechanism is called compensatory evolution. It occurs when an organism makes up for the cost of a new mutation by compensating with another mutation rather than reverting back to the earlier drug-sensitive form. Such mechanisms have been found for mutations that would otherwise decrease bacterial synthesis of important molecules, except that additional mutations restore production levels while still conferring resistance. Such compensation has been found in persistently drug-resistant strains of *Salmonella, Staphylococcus, Step. pneumonia,* and *M. tuberculosis* (Andersson and Hughes 2011).

Thirdly, two or more resistance genes may be closely linked together such that, even in the absence of one antibiotic, the presence of another antibiotic may tend to keep both genes around. Such is the case for certain strains of *Pseudomonas aeruginosa* known to cause pneumonia in mechanically ventilated patients. Here, two genes are closely linked, each conferring resistance to a different class of antibiotics, such that both persist in the presence of only one of these kinds of drugs (Reinhardt et al. 2007).

Finally, it should be noted that even when the evolution of reversal is possible, the process can be very slow if the costs of resistance are relatively cheap. One experiment predicted that it would take a tetracycline-resistant E. coli population a year and a half to replace 99.9 per cent of its members with drug-sensitive revertants, assuming that the resistance only resulted in a 0.7 per cent reduction in growth (Andersson and Hughes 2011). This last mechanism underscores the impact of small differences on the direction and rate of evolutionary change. We can consider the impact of environmental changes within and surrounding human hosts just as we can consider the impact of genetic changes on the pathogens. Both can have significant impacts on the persistence or reversal of antibiotic resistance.

At present, the future does not look good for the prevention of antibiotic resistance. The genetic adaptations of pathogens have greatly outpaced the cultural adaptations of their human hosts. Industrial agriculture has permeated our global environment with antibiotics. The consumption of these antibiotics has transformed our bodily flora into reservoirs for drug-resistance genes, which we can pass on to other pathogens. And the most vulnerable of our human communities—the elderly, the impoverished, and the chronically sick—are gateways and incubators for the emergence of new, drug-resistant strains of human pathogens. Laurie Garrett, a Pulitzer Prize-winning health writer and trained biologist, predicts that we are heading back to the times of our recent ancestors in what she calls "the post-antibiotic era" (1994).

That said, antibiotics are not likely to disappear soon, and they are not likely to disappear all at once. Even if we finally run out of safe antibiotic options, we could take solace in the lessons of the Second Epidemiological Transition, when we made our greatest strides in the reduction of infectious diseases prior to the availability of such medicines. We could then see the evolution of resistance as a wake-up call for better health practices, programs, and policies. Certainly we should continue to work on new medicines, and we should do everything possible to slow down the evolution of resistance, but we should also apply the ancient and recurring lessons for human health in our current modes of subsistence, settlement, and social organization. Resistance may still be inevitable, but it need not be catastrophic.

7

Conclusion

This book has sought to dispel three major myths about emerging infectious diseases. The first is that emerging infections are a new phenomenon. On the contrary, we have seen evidence for the first rise of acute and virulent human infections with the advent of agriculture 10 000 years ago. Moreover, we know that the evolution of drug resistance is far older insofar as microbes have been using these mechanisms to defend against each other for at least a billion years. Accounting for these time lines, it could be argued that there are no truly emerging infections today, only re-emerging infections.

The second myth is that emerging and re-emerging infections are primarily natural or spontaneous phenomena. Instead, we have examined how our species has strongly influenced the evolution of our microbial neighbors (and tenants)—pathogenic or otherwise—by the ways that we live with each other, and the ways we live with the plants and animals around us. In this age of Germ Theory, it is no small irony that the same professionals who can describe the detailed molecular mechanisms of pathogens—the *hows* of human infection—will nevertheless resort to the old Doctrine of Spontaneous Generation when trying to explain *why* these mechanisms evolved to make us sick in the first place. To improve this explanation, an expanded framework of epidemiological transitions helps complement the microscopic perspective with a macroscopic perspective. Both are necessary to achieve a comprehensive understanding of emerging infectious diseases.

The third myth is that the disease determinants of our past are qualitatively different from those of the present. To be sure, we live in a very different world today than that of our ancient ancestors. But we have seen throughout this book that the major themes governing our susceptibility to infectious diseases today are essentially the same as those of our ancient past: they are merely intensified by our massive populations, our cities, and the technologies now at our disposal. This continuity brings an additional challenge to the old adage that "those who forget history are doomed to repeat it." Here, we must first become aware of history before we can hope to remember it.

Fernand Braudel, one of the founding historians of the Annales School, states that "history may be divided into three movements: what moves rapidly, what moves slowly, and what appears not to move at all" (Braudel 1972:8). Indeed, some histories are so long that we are unaware of their existence. Like continents, they appear to be permanent fixtures, even as

An Unnatural History of Emerging Infections. First Edition. Ron Barrett and George J. Armelagos
© Ron Barrett and George J. Armelagos 2013. Published 2013 by Oxford University Press.

they shift and shape one another, traveling the world and colliding over great stretches of time. Then, in a single day, an earthquake happens, a tsunami lands, and a nuclear reactor breaks down. We are spellbound by these sudden disasters, having ignored the larger and slower forces leading up to their occurrence. Historians of the Annales School refer to these latter processes as the *longue durée*.

The three Epidemiological Transitions presented in this book provide ample material for *longue durée* analysis. Here, we have examined events that have largely escaped historical attention but turned out to have profound effects on human health: changes in human food production and human reproduction, changes in social hierarchies and social densities, changes in climates, cultures, and physical constitutions. To be fair, some of these events were deeply buried in human prehistory, uncovered only by the painstaking methods of the archeologist or physical anthropologist. But many events occurred and recurred in plain sight of authors who could have recorded them, but focused instead on great battles and the lives of the rich and powerful. All the while, the human determinants of human infections were camouflaged by their scope and scale.

In the Third Transition of the present day, it is ironic that we pay much more attention to the roles of invisibly small creatures than the plainly visible ones that are more than a trillion times larger. The medical historian, William McNeill, used the terms *microparasite* and *macroparasite* to compare the behaviors of disease-causing microbes and disease-causing humans (McNeill 1976). Both make their livings at the hosts' expense, and the interactions between them produce sickness. Yet unlike the microparasite, who blindly adapts to its surroundings by random changes, the macroparasite adapts by intentional changes—even if these changes produce unintended consequences.

Because of human intention, the origins of human epidemics could not be called "natural" in the same way that we would describe the origins of earthquakes or tsunamis. Instead, they are more like those of nuclear reactors, unnatural products of human artifice. Still, it is easy to see the epidemics as natural disasters because pathogens are living creatures, and it is often easier—psychologically and socially—to observe their molecular influences than it is to observe their human influences. This is especially the case when human influences take the form of human inequalities. Returning to the earthquake analogy, it would seem at first glance that the 2010 quake in Haiti was a "natural disaster." But a different picture emerges if we compare statistics from the Haitian earthquake with one that occurred in the United States:

2010 Haiti: 7.0 Richter at the epicenter, 16 miles from a major urban center, 220 000 deaths.

1989 California (USA): 6.8 Richter at the epicenter, 16 miles from a major urban center, 63 deaths.

The natural characteristics of these two earthquakes were quite similar. Their intensities were comparable, even for a logarithmic scale, and their epicenters were the same distance from a major urban area: Port-au-Prince in Haiti, San Francisco in California. Yet the Haitian earthquake resulted in 3500-fold greater mortality than the Californian quake—an enormous difference that cannot be explained by natural factors. However, it can be explained on a similar scale of economic differences as measured by instruments such as the Human Development

Index, by which the United States ranked fourth while Haiti ranked 145th out of 169 countries. Haiti is the poorest country in the western hemisphere, and in Port-au-Prince, 86 per cent of the population lived in slum conditions before the quake. Only half the population had access to toilets and only a third had access to running water (Farmer 2011). Given these conditions, it is not surprising that the earthquake would be followed by epidemic infections, including drug-resistant cholera, for which mortality would remain high for many years. The earth-quake itself was a natural event, but the long-standing reasons for its devastation and after-math were highly unnatural.

The primary purpose of this *Unnatural History* is to reveal the macroscopic determinants of human infections just as the germ theorists once revealed their microscopic determi-nants. We certainly do not dismiss the importance of Germ Theory. Rather, our approach has been one of both seed and soil, acknowledging the importance of pathogens while stressing their evolution in response to human activities: the ways we feed ourselves, the ways we populate and live together, and the ways we relate to each other for better and worse. Like the Annales historians, we have tried to present these issues across greater stretches of time, from the late Paleolithic to the early 21st century, so we can see the recur-ring nature of these determinants.

7.1 Subsistence: Then and Now

In Chapter 1, we argued that modern humans are essentially "stone agers living in the fast lane" (Eaton et al. 1988a). Because of the slow pace of human biological evolution, we are physiologically no different than our Paleolithic ancestors, even if our lifestyles and sur-roundings are radically different. Thus, having examined the protective role of nutrition against human infections today, we could infer the same protective role in our ancestors, who must have had diverse sources of essential nutrients, even if they sometimes dealt with toxins and seasonal shortages. Then, after the intensification of agriculture reduced dietary diversity, we saw skeletal evidence of increasing nutritional deficiencies and acute infections.

Jared Diamond once said that agriculture was the "worst mistake in the human race" (1987: 86). This may have been an exaggeration, but the nutritional impacts of this subsistence change had a dramatic effect on our susceptibility to what were then novel, acute, and viru-lent infections. Moreover, our domestication of animals for food and farm work brought us into close proximity with zoonotic pathogens, presenting them with repeated opportunities to make incursions into undernourished human populations, the so-called "viral chatter" that we observe with new infections today. As these zoonoses evolved human-to-human transmissibility, they became the first truly "emerging" infectious diseases in the human race: the domesticated pathogens of the First Epidemiological Transition.

Again, we saw the role of changing subsistence in the Second Epidemiological Transition. Here, improvements in farming and food distribution brought better nutrition to affluent societies that were early adopters of the Industrial Revolution. While improved nutrition may not have been the sole or even chief determinant of mortality decline, it was undoubtedly one of several major factors that preceded the development of antimicrobial drugs. The latter were more important in the Second Transitions of the developing world. This was partly due to timing, as most of these transitions occurred after antibiotic medicines became available. But it was also due to the fact that the developing world had not experienced the same degree of improvements in living conditions enjoyed by their more affluent neighbors. As a consequence, the impoverished majority of the developing world found themselves in a worst-of-both-worlds scenario, with sharp rises in chronic degenerative diseases, and only modest if any declines in acute infectious diseases. When these diseases, returned to haunt the affluent world, they became known as "re-emerging" infections—new labels for old problems.

Food production was industrialized on a massive scale in the years leading up to the Third Epidemiological Transition. Food animals became urbanized, densely stacked under stressful conditions in large-scale production facilities. These populations served as reservoirs for new strains of old infections, broadly disseminated through distribution networks for supermarkets and fast-food restaurants, not to mention the water supplies downstream of their artificial habitats. To make matters worse, the use of sub-therapeutic antibiotics as animal growth-agents has promoted the evolution and transmission, not only of drug-resistant organisms, but also the genes responsible for these characteristics. In this manner, resistance has been transmitted back and forth between pathogens and normal flora of the human gut. Finally, with the expansion of human societies into receding wilderness areas, practices such as bushmeat hunting have brought humans into contact with zoonotic pathogens that had been infecting nonhuman primates, our closest evolutionary relatives with whom we have much in common, including susceptibility to many of the same infections. Our ancient ancestors probably faced the same risks, but they were not as interconnected as we are today.

7.2 Settlement: Then and Now

The earliest form of human settlement was hardly settled at all. For a hundred millennia, *Homo sapiens* lived as nomads, broadly and thinly scattered throughout the world in small groups comprised of no more than a few dozen people. Even earlier, our hominid precursors lived this way for more than 4 million years. All told, the vast majority of human evolution has occurred while on the move. This level of mobility and group size could not have supported the sustained human-to-human transmission of acute infectious diseases. Chronic infections may well have been a problem, especially the less virulent parasites we inherited from our pre-human ancestors and picked up as "souvenirs" in the course of our travels. But most of the human infections we know today would have quickly burned out among our nomadic ancestors, spreading no further than to a few human groups.

To have remained unsettled for so long, our nomadic ancestors had to keep their group sizes small. They could have accomplished this in at least one of two ways: first, by maintaining very low or zero population growth through relatively balanced birth and death rates; and second, by fissioning oversized groups into small ones and then expanding into different territories. However, both strategies have their perturbations and limits, and these probably contributed to the crises that preceded the Agricultural Revolutions. Nevertheless, the lesson remains that human settlement is closely tied to human demographics. The same could be said for our modes of subsistence and social organization, as we have seen throughout this book, but settlement is a good base for demographics insofar as it has us thinking about how many people live where and under what conditions. These latter factors have strongly determined our susceptibility to infectious diseases.

Settlement was a major factor in the First Transition, when our ancient ancestors stopped moving around and starting farming in earnest. Human populations increased. Domestic animal populations increased. And both lived in much greater densities in the same locations, thereby supporting the sustained transmission of acute infections. These densities rose much higher with the development of towns and cities, which became interlinked through long-distance trade networks between expanding empires and state-level societies. These were the halcyon years for many plagues of many human pathogens.

We saw how changing modes of settlement could have contributed to the mortality declines of the Second Transition. The housing reforms in late 19th-century Europe may have helped, but more likely contributions were made by the development of water and waste infrastructures to meet the demands of growing urban populations—at least, in economically better developed societies. For the rest of the world, the rapid urbanization of poor societies has presented major opportunities for the incubation and spread of new, virulent, and drug-resistant infections of the Third Transition. We now live in a world where the majority of 7 billion people live in urban areas, and all our settlements are situated in a global network for the movement of nearly everybody and the exchange of nearly everything, including of course, our microbial pathogens. Our recent patterns of human settlement have created a single, global disease ecology.

7.3 Social Organization: Then and Now

A recurring theme throughout this book has been that new and drug-resistant pathogens first enter human populations through their most vulnerable members. This makes sense, given that most of our infections originated from zoonotic pathogens for which the evolution of human-to-human transmission was a stepwise process, and that this process was even more incremental for multi-drug-resistant strains. The first and smallest of these increments is the infection of human hosts who are undernourished, overstressed, and compromised by existing infections or chronic diseases. Such hosts are most likely to be poor and under 5 years of age, or increasingly, poor and over 60 years of age. In this manner, the impoverished majority of our species are unwilling gateways, or sentinels, for the emerging infections associated with the Third Epidemiological Transition. They can also serve as reservoirs for amplification of these infections, both in number and virulence, as well as their persistence over time.

We know from many ethnographic studies that most contemporary foraging societies have social structures that are simpler and more egalitarian than their sedentary counterparts (Marlowe 2005). This is not to suggest that all foraging societies are free from violence and oppression, or that there are not important gender-based inequalities within them. But further social differences and leadership structures are cumbersome and unnecessary for the functioning of small groups, and without these structures, there is little chance for the unequal distribution of resources. This is once again reflected in the ethnographic record, in which there is a common theme of resource sharing and social sanctions against people having more than their share (Kelly 1995; Lee and Daly 1999).

The Agricultural Revolution brought radical changes to our resource distribution patterns. We saw this in the burial sites of ancient societies during their transitions from foraging to agriculture. People often die as they lived, and we have seen this reflected in people's graves. In the earlier stages of their agricultural transition, ancient societies buried their dead with similar artifacts in similar graves. Then, with the intensification of agriculture, differences arose in the quality of artifacts and graves, indicating greater socio-economic differences. It is not surprisingly that the skeletons of higher-status people show fewer signs of disease than those of lower-status people. What may be surprising, however, is that these are the first empirical signs of social and health inequalities in the archaeological record. We do not have evidence for major inequalities prior to the Agricultural Revolution; it could therefore be argued therefore that such differences have not been a natural constant of the human condition.

Moving from the Agricultural Revolution to the Industrial Revolution, the Second Epidemiological Transition presents both positive and negative examples of the links between socio-economic differences and infectious diseases. We have found positive examples within the more affluent societies that initially underwent the Second Transition, where declining mortality was often correlated with indicators of reduced health differences (however modest) among people of all social classes (Hauspie et al. 1997; McKeown 1988). These correlations make sense when we consider that infectious diseases had been the primary causes of death and reducing the risk of infection among the poorer classes also reduced the risk of infection for everyone else.

Unfortunately, the negative examples of differences and disease occurred at much larger scales during the latter decades of the Second Transition. While poorer societies also benefitted from declining infections, most of these improvements occurred much later and leveled off much sooner than in wealthier nations. Yet at the same time, poorer societies have had to contend with rapid increases in chronic diseases and rapidly aging populations—the same health challenges as the affluent world but with fewer resources to deal with them. Lastly, mortality declines in the developing world have been, and continue to be, much more dependent on antimicrobial medicines than in the developed world. This is a particularly troubling problem when we consider rise of drug-resistant infections in the Third Epidemiological Transition.

7.4 Moving Beyond the Third Transition

Today, the globalization of human infections means that the health risks among the poor increase the health risks for everyone else. While people may debate the "trickle-down" effects of the global marketplace, there is no question that human pathogens are "trickling up" at a much faster rate. This reality brings us back to the very first point in this book: that microbes are the ultimate critics of modernity. But criticism should not beget fatalism, nor should the poor be blamed for the shortcomings of larger societies. If anything, our awareness of these global issues should raise our senses of individual and collective responsibility.

An expanded framework of epidemiological transitions can do more than expand awareness. It can inform policies and programs aimed at improving the prevention and advanced detection of human infections. For instance, if we understand the common and long-standing determinants of many infections and other health problems, then we can organize our health efforts around these fewer, upstream determinants instead of dealing with many more downstream consequences after they have already occurred. Denis Burkitt, an Irish surgeon who drew important contrasts between preventable health problems in Africa and Europe, summed up the situation in very concrete terms:

> Western doctors are like poor plumbers. They treat a splashing tube by cleaning up the water. These plumbers are extremely apt at drying up the water, constantly inventing new, expensive, and refined methods of drying up water. Somebody should teach them how to close the tap. (Burkitt 1979:16).

Closing the tap entails closing the gap in healthy living and health care within and between human populations. It entails a redoubling of the positive efforts that brought the Second Transition to many societies until all societies reach similarly low levels of infectious disease mortality. History shows that great gains were made with fewer resources than we have today. Now, our global economy has given us greater means, and our global diseases have given us more reasons to tackle this problem than ever before. Better physical health also entails better fiscal health for all nations around the world. Whether for survival, prosperity, or ethics, the argument for improving health amongst all populations should hold sway across a broad spectrum of political philosophies.

Understanding the convergence of disease patterns can also inform greater efficiency in the organization and delivery of health services. Case in point, the US Centers for Disease Control recognizes the syndemic nature of AIDS, STDs, TB, and hepatitis epidemics. With syndemics in mind, it has recently brought together divisions and branches that once addressed these diseases separately (<http://www.cdc.gov/nchhstp/programintegration>, last accessed October 26, 2012). This kind of program integration is often referred to as a "horizontal approach" to public health, in contrast to vertical programs that traditionally focused on single diseases.

Horizontal approaches minimize redundancies, promote collaborations, and perhaps most importantly, focus more attention on the common determinants of multiple diseases (Nichter 2008). Inevitably, most of these determinants are social determinants, the same themes we have been exploring throughout this book. Let us hope such programs become pandemic, and that they spread across all manner of health challenges. We can then write about the positive lessons of the next Epidemiological Transition.

References

Ackerknecht, E. H. 1948/2009. Anticontagionism between 1821 and 1867. *International Journal of Epidemiology*, 38, 7–21.

Alexander, D. J. 2000. A review of avian influenza in different bird species. *Veterinary Microbiology*, 74, 3–13.

Ames, K. M. 2004. Supposing Hunter-Gatherer variability. *American Antiquity*, 69, 364–74.

Amyes, S. 2001. *Magic Bullets, Lost Horizons: The Rise and Fall of Antibiotics*, New York: Taylor & Francis.

Anderson, R. M., Fraser, C., Ghani, A. C., Donnelly, C. A., Riley, S., Ferguson, N. M., Leung, G. M., Lam, T. H., and Hedley, A. J. 2004. Epidemiology, Transmission Dynamics, and Control of SARS: The 2002–2003 Epidemic. *Philosophical Transactions of the Royal Society of London: Series B-Biological Sciences*, 359, 1091–105.

Anderson, R. M. and May, R. M. 1986. The Invasion, Peristence and Spread of Infectious Diseases within Animal and Plant Communities. *Philosophical Transactions of the Royal Society of London Series B-Biological Sciences*, 314, 533–70.

Andersson, D. I. and Hughes, D. 2011. Persistence of antibiotic resistance in bacterial populations. *Fems Microbiology Reviews*, 35, 901–11.

Andrade, L. H., Wang, Y. P., Andreoni, S., Silveira, C. M., Alexandrino-Silva, C., Siu, E. R., Nishimura, R., Anthony, J. C., Gattaz, W. F., and Kessler, R. C. 2012. Mental Disorders in Megacities: Findings from the São Paulo Megacity Mental Health Survey, Brazil. *PLoS ONE*, 7, e31879.

Angel, J. L. 1984. Health as a crucial factor in the changes from hunting to developed farming in the eastern Mediterranean. *In:* Cohen, M. N. and Armelagos, G. J. (eds) *Paleopathology at the Origins of Agriculture*, Orlando, FL: Academic Press.

Armelagos, G. J. 2010. The Evolution of the Brain and the Determinants of Food Choice. *Journal of Anthropological Research*, 66, 161–86.

Armelagos, G. J. and Baker, B. J. 1988. The Origin and Antiquity of Syphilis. *Current Anthropology*, 29, 703–37.

Armelagos, G. J. and Brown, P. J. 2002. The Body as Evidence; The Body of Evidence. *In:* Steckel, R. and Rose, J. (eds), *Backbone of History: Health and Nutrition in the Western Hemisphere*, New York: Cambridge University Press.

Armelagos, G. J., Brown, P. J., and Turner, B. 2005. Evolutionary, historical and political economic perspectives on health and disease. *Social Science & Medicine*, 61, 755–65.

Armelagos, G. J., Goodman, A. H., and Jacobs, K. 1991. The Origins of Agriculture: Population Growth During a Period of Declining Health. *Cultural Change and Population Growth: An Evolutionary Perspective a Special Issue of Population and Environment*, 13, 9–22.

Armelagos, G. J. and Harper, K. N. 2009. Emerging Infectious Diseases, Urbanization and Globalization in the Time of Global Warming. *In:* Cockerham, W. C. (ed.) *The Blackwell Companion to Medical Sociology,* Hoboken, NJ: Wiley Publishing.

Armelagos, G. J., Kohlbacher, K., Collins, K. R., Cook, J., and Karfield-Daugherty, M. 2001. Tetracycline consumption in prehistory. *In:* Nelson, M., Hillen, W., and Greenwald, R. A. (eds) *Tetracyclines in Biology, Chemistry and Medicine,* Basil: Birkhauser Verlag AG.

Asher, M. I. 2011. Urbanisation, asthma and allergies. *Thorax,* 66, 1025–6.

Audette, R. V. and Gilchrist, T. 1995. *NeanderThin: Eat Like a Caveman to Achieve A Lean Strong Healthy Body,* New York: St. Martin's Press.

Ayele, W., Neill, S., Zinsstag, J., Weiss, M., and Pavlik, I. 2004. Bovine Tuberculosis: An Old Disease but a New Threat to Africa. *The International Journal of Tuberculosis and Lung Disease,* 8, 924–37.

Bager, F., Aarestrup, F. M., and Wegener, H. C. 2000. Dealing with antimicrobial resistance—the Danish experience. *Canadian Journal of Animal Science,* 80, 223–8.

Barker, D. J. P. 2004. The Developmental Origins of Adult Disease. *Journal of the American College of Nutrition,* 23, 589S–95S.

Barker, D. J. P. 2007. The Origins of the Developmental Origins Theory. *Journal of Internal Medicine,* 261, 412–17.

Barnes, D. S. 1995. *The Making of a Social Disease; Tuberculosis in Nineteenth-Century France,* Berkeley: University of California Press.

Barrett, R. 2006a. Dark winter and the spring of 1972: Deflecting the social lessons of smallpox. *Medical Anthropology,* 25, 171–91.

Barrett, R. 2006b. Human Ecology and False Allegations: The 1994 Plague in Western India. *In:* Lavoy, P. and Clunan, A. (eds) *Terrorism, War, or Disease? Unraveling the Use of Biological Weapons,* Stanford, CA: Stanford University Press.

Barrett, Ron 2008. *Aghor Medicine: Pollution, Death, and Healing in Northern India,* Berkeley: University of California Press.

Barrett, R. 2010. Avian Influenza and the Third Epidemiological Transition. *In:* Herring, A. and Swedlund, A. C. (eds) *Plagues and Epidemics: Infected Spaces Past and Present,* New York: Bergin.

Barrett, R., Kuzawa, C. W., Mcdade, T., and Armelagos, G. J. 1998. Emerging infectious disease and the third epidemiological transition. *In:* Durham, W. (ed.) *Annual Review Anthropology,* 27, 247–71.

Bassett, E., Keith, M., Armelagos, G. J., Martin, D., and Villanueva, A. 1980. Tetracycline Labeled Human Bone from Prehistoric Sudanese Nubia (A.D. 350). *Science,* 1532–1534.

Berlin, B. 1992. *Ethnobiological Classification: Principles of Categorization of Plants in Traditional Societies,* Princeton, NJ: Princeton University Press.

Binford, L. 2001. *Constructing Frames of Reference: An Analytical Method for Archaeological Theory Building Using Hunter-Gatherer and Environmental Data Sets,* Berkeley, CA: University of California Press.

Black, F. L. 1975. Infectious Diseases in Primitive Societies. *Science,* 187, 515–18.

Black, F. L. 1980. Modern Isolated Pre-Agricultural Populations as a Source of Information on Prehistoric Epidemic Patterns. *In:* Stanley, N. F. and Joske, R. A. (eds) *Changing Disease Patterns and Human Behavior,* London: Academic Press.

Black, F. L. 1992. Why Did They Die? *Science,* 258, 1739–40.

Bloom, D. E. and Canning, D. 2007. Mortality Traps and the Dynamics of Health Transitions. *Proceedings of the National Academy of Sciences,* 104, 16044–9.

Boni, M. F., Gog, J. R., Andreasen, V., and Christiansen, F. B. 2004. Influenza drift and epidemic size: the race between generating and escaping immunity. *Theoretical Population Biology,* 65, 179–91.

Bozzoli, C., Deaton, A., and Quintana-Domeque, C. 2009. Adult height and childhood disease. *Demography,* 46, 647–69.

Bradley, D. 1993. Environmental and Health Problems of Developing Countries. *1993 Environmental Change and Human Health,* Chichester: Ciba Foundation.

Braidwood, L. S. 1983. *Prehistoric archeology along the Zagros Flanks,* Chicago, IL, Oriental Institute of the University of Chicago.

Braidwood, R. J. 1967. *Prehistoric men,* Glenview, IL, Scott Foresman.

Braudel, F. 1972. *The Mediterranean and the Mediterranean World in the Age of Phillip II,* New York, NY: Simon & Schuster.

Bray, R. S. 1996. *Armies of Pestilence: The Impact of Disease on History,* Cambridge, UK, James Clark & Co.

Brock, T. D. 1988. *Robert Koch: A life in medicine and bacteriology,* Washington, DC: American Society for Microbiology.

Broughton, G. I. I., Janis, J. E., and Attinger, C. E. 2006. A brief history of wound care. *Plastic and reconstructive surgery,* 117, 6S–11S.

Brown, K. 2004. The history of penicillin from discovery to the drive to production. *Pharmaceutical Historian,* 34, 37–43.

Brown, R.A. and Armelagos, G.J. 2001. Apportionment of Racial Diversity: A Review. *Evolutionary Anthropology,* 10, 34–40.

Bryce, J., Boschi-Pinto, C., Shibuya, K., and Black, R. E. 2005. WHO estimates of the causes of death in children. *The Lancet,* 365, 1147–52.

Buikstra, J. E. 1984. The Lower Illinois River Region: A Prehistoric Context for the Study of Ancient Health and Diet. In Paleopathology at the Origins of Agriculture. *In:* Cohen, M. N.

and Armelagos, G. J. (eds) *Paleopathology at the Origins of Agriculture*, Orlando, FL: Academic Press.

Burkitt, D. 1979. *Don't Forget Fibre in Your Diet*, London, Collins.

Burnet, M. 1962. *Natural History of Infectious Disease*, Cambridge, UK, Cambridge University Press.

Burnett, J. 1991. Housing and the Decline in Mortality. *In:* Schofield, R., Reher, D., and Bideau, A. (eds) *The Decline of Mortality in Europe*, Oxford: Oxford University Press.

Caldwell, J. C. 1976. Toward a Restatement of Demographic Transition Theory. *Popuation and Development Review*, 2, 321-66.

Centers for Disease Control and Prevention. 1981. Kaposi's Sarcoma and Pneumocystis Pneumonia among Homosexual Men- New York City and California. *Morbidity and Mortality Weekly Report*, 30, 305-8.

Centers for Disease Control and Prevention. 2011. *Known Cases and Outbreaks of Ebola Hemorrhagic Fever in Chronological Order*, <http://www.cdc.gov/ncidod/dvrd/spb/mnpages/dispages/ebola/ebolatable.pdf> last accessed October 30, 2011.

Chan, J. W. M., Ng, C. K., Chan, Y. H., Mok, T. Y. W., Lee, S., Chu, S. Y. Y., Law, W. L., Lee, M. P., and Li, P. C. K. 2003. Short term outcome and risk factors for adverse clinical outcomes in adults with severe acute respiratory syndrome (SARS). *Thorax*, 58, 686-9.

Chandra, R. K. 1997. Nutrition and the Immune System: An Introduction. *American Journal of Clinical Nutrition*, 66, 460S-463S.

Cheung, C. Y., Poon, L. L. M., Lau, A. S., Luk, W., Lau, Y. L., Shortridge, K. F., Gordon, S., Guan, Y., and Peiris, J. S. M. 2002. Induction of proinflammatory cytokines in human macrophages by influenza A (H5N1) viruses: a mechanism for the unusual severity of human disease? *Lancet*, 360, 1831-7.

Clemente, J. C., Ursell, L. K., Parfrey, L. W., and Knight, R. 2012. The Impact of the Gut Microbiota on Human Health: An Integrated View. *Cell*, 148, 1258-70.

Coale, A. J. 1974. The History of the Human Population. *Scientific American*, 231, 40-51.

Cockburn, T. A. 1967. The evolution of human infectious diseases. *In:* Cockburn, T. A. (ed.) *Infectious Diseases: Their Evolution and Eradication*, Springfield, IL: Charles C. Thomas.

Cockburn, T. A. 1971. Infectious disease in ancient populations. *Current Anthropology*, 12, 45-62.

Cohen, H. W., Gould, R. M., and Sidel, V. W. 2004. The Pitfalls of Bioterrorism Preparedness: the Anthrax and Smallpox Experiences. *American Journal of Public Health*, 94, 1667-71.

Cohen, M. N. 1977. *The Food Crisis in Prehistory: Overpopulation and the Origins of Agriculture*, New Haven Conn., Yale University Press.

Cohen, M. N. 2009. Introduction: Rethinking the Origins of Agriculture. *Current Anthropology*, 50, 591-5.

Cohen, M. N. and Armelagos, G. J. (eds) 1984. *Paleopathology at the Origins of Agriculture,* Orlando, FL: Academic Press.

Cole, T. J. 2000. Secular Trends in Growth. *Proceedings of the Nutrition Society,* 59, 317-24.

Cordain, L. 2002. *The PaleoDiet: Lose Weight and Get Healthy by Eating the Food You Were Designed to Eat,* New York, NY: J. Wiley.

Cordain, L., Miller, J. B., Eaton, S. B., Mann, N., Holt, S. H. A., and Speth, J. D. 2000. Plant-Animal Subsistence Ratios and Macronutrient Energy Estimations in Worldwide Hunter-Gatherer Diets. *American Journal of Clinical Nutrition,* 71, 682-92.

Cottingham, K. L., Chiavelli, D. A., and Taylor, R. K. 2003. Environmental microbe and human pathogen: the ecology and microbiology of *Vibrio Cholerae. Frontiers in Ecology and the Environment,* 1, 80-6.

Crosby, A. W. 1976. Virgin soil epidemics as a factor in the aboriginal depopulation in America. *The William and Mary Quarterly,* 33, 289-99.

Crosby, A. W. 1989. *America's Forgotten Pandemic: The Influenza of 1918,* Cambridge, UK: Cambridge University Press.

Crosby, A. W. 2003. *The Columbian Exchange: Biological and Cultural Consequences of 1492,* Wesport, Praeger.

D'costa, V. M., King, C. E., Kalan, L., Morar, M., Sung, W. W. L., Schwarz, C., Froese, D., Zazula, G., Calmels, F., Debruyne, R., Golding, G. B., Poinar, H. N., and Wright, G. D. 2011. Antibiotic resistance is ancient. *Nature,* 477, 457-61.

Davis, M. 2006. *The Monster at our Door: The Global Threat of Avian Flu,* New York, NY: Owl Books.

Diamond, J. 1987. The Worst Mistake in the History of the Human Race. *Discover,* New York, NY: Family Media.

Diamond, M. and Stone, M. 1981. Nightingale on Quetelet. *Journal of the Royal Statistical Society. Series A (General),* 144, 66-79.

Dickinson, E. 1896. Time and Eternity, Poem 24. *Poems of Emily Dickinson,* Boston, MA: Robert Brother.

Dinh, P. N., Long, H. T., Tien, N. T. K., Hien, N. T., Mai, L. T. Q., Phong, L. H., Tuan, L. V., Tan, H. V., Nguyen, N. B., Van Tu, P., and Phuong, N. T. M. 2006. Risk factors for human infection with avian influenza A H5N1, Vietnam, 2004. *Emerging Infectious Diseases,* 12, 1841-7.

Dobell, C. 1932. *Antony van Leeuwenhoek and His "Little Animals,"* New York, NY: Dover Publications.

Dobyns, H. F. 1993. Disease Transfer at Contact. *Annual Review of Anthropology,* 22, 273-91.

Dowell, S. F., Mukunu, R., Ksiazek, T. G., Khan, A. S., Rollin, P. E., Peters, C. J., and Commission Lutte Epidemies, K. 1999. Transmission of Ebola hemorrhagic fever: A study of risk factors in family members, Kikwit, Democratic Republic of the Congo, 1995. *Journal of Infectious Diseases,* 179, S87-91.

Dubos, R. J. 1959. *Mirage of Health: Utopias, Progress, and Biological Change,* New York, NY: Harper and Brothers.

Dye, C. 2008. Health and Urban Living. *Science,* 319, 766–9.

Eaton, S. B. and Eaton III, S. B. 2000. Paleolithic vs. Modern Diets: Selected Pathophysiological Implications. *European Journal of Nutrition,* 39, 67–70.

Eaton, S. B. and Konner, M. 1985. Paleolithic nutrition. A consideration of its nature and current implications. *New England Journal of Medicine,* 312, 283–9.

Eaton, S. B., Konner, M., and Shostak, M. 1988a. Stone agers in the fast lane: chronic degenerative diseases in evolutionary perspective. *American Journal of Medicine,* 84, 739–49.

Eaton, S. B., Shostak, M., and Konner, M. 1988b. *The Paleolithic Prescription: A Program of Diet & Exercise and a Design for Living,* New York, NY: Harper and Row.

Eaton, S. B., Pike, M. C., Short, R. V., Lee, N. C., Trussell, J., Hatcher, R. A., Wood, J. W, Worthman, C. M., Jones, N. G. B., Konner, M. J., Hill, K. R., Bailey, R., and Hurtado, A. M. 1994. Women's Reproductive Cancers in Evolutionary Context. *Quarterly Review of Biology,* Vol. 69, 353–67.

Ebenstein, A. 2012. The Consequences of Industrialization: Evidence from Water Pollution and Digestive Cancers in China. *The Review of Economics and Statistics,* 94, 186–201.

Ehreth, J. 2003. The Global Value of Vaccination. *Vaccine,* 21, 596–600.

Ellen, R. 1995. Science or Molecule Hunting? *Anthropology Today,* 11, 1–2.

Endicott, K. L. 1999. Gender Relations in Hunter-Gatherer Societies. *In:* Panter-Brick, C., Layton, R. and Rowley-Conwy, P. (eds) *The Cambridge Encyclopedia of Hunter-Gatherers,* Cambridge UK: Cambridge University Press.

Etkin, N. L. 1996. Ethnopharmacology: The Conjunction of Medical Ethnography and the Biology of Therapeutic Action. *In:* Sargent, C. F. and Johnson, T. M. (eds) *Medical Anthropology: Contemporary Theory and Method,* Westport, CT: Praeger.

Euling, S. Y., Selevan, S. G., Pescovitz, O. H., and Skakkabaek, N. E. 2008. Role of Environmental Factors in the Timing of Puberty. *Pediatrics,* 121, S167–71.

Ewald, P. W. 1983. Host-Parasite Relations, Vectors, and the Evolution of Disease Severity *Annual Review of Ecology and Systematics,* 14, 465–85.

Ewald, P. W. 1994. *Evolution of Infectious Disease,* New York, Oxford University Press.

Eyler, J. M. 1979. *Victorian Social Medicine: the Ideas and Methods of William Farr,* Baltimore, MD: Johns Hopkins University Press.

Farmer, P. 1992. *AIDS and Accusation: Haiti and the Geography of Blame,* Berkeley, CA: University of California Press.

Farmer, P. 1996. Social Inequalities and Emerging Infectious Diseases. *Emerging Infectious Diseases,* 2, 259–69.

Farmer, P. 1997. Social scientists and the new tuberculosis. *Social Science & Medicine,* 44, 347–58.

Farmer, P. 2011. *Haiti After the Earthquake,* New York, Public Affairs Books.

Fenner, F., Henderson, D. A., Arita, I., Jezek, Z., and Ladnyi, I. D. 1988. *Smallpox and its Eradication,* Geneva: World Health Organization.

Field, C. J., Johnson, I. R., and Schley, P. D. 2002. Nutrients and their role in host resistance to infection. *Journal of Leukocyte Biology,* 71, 16–32.

Fierer, N., Hamady, M., Lauber, C. L., and Knight, R. 2008. The influence of sex, handedness, and washing on the diversity of hand surface bacteria. *Proceedings of the National Academy of Sciences of the United States of America,* 105, 17994–9.

Foege, W. H., Millar, J. D., and Henderson, D. A. 1975. Smallpox Eradication in West and Central Africa. *Bulletin of the World Health Organization,* 52, 209–22.

Food and Agriculture Organization of the United Nations 2012. The State of Food Insecurity in the World, 2012. Rome: Food and Agriculture Organization of the United Nations.

Fowler, M. L. 1997. *The Cahokia Atlas: A Historical Atlas of Cahokia Archaeology,* Urbana, IL: University of Illinois Press.

Fracastoro, H. F. G. 1530. *Syphilidis, sive Morbi Gallici,* Lipsiae: Leopoldum.

Froment, A. 2001. Evolutionary Biology and Health of Hunter-Gatherer Populations. *In:* Panter-Brick, C., Layton, R. and Rowley-Conwy, P. (eds) *Hunter-Gatherers: An Interdisciplinary Perspective.* Cambridge UK: Cambridge University Press.

Furuse, Y., Suzuki, A., and Oshitani, H. 2010. Origin of Measles Virus: Divergence from Rinderpest Virus between the 11th and 12th Centuries. *Virology Journal,* 7, 52–5.

Galea, S. 2011. The urban brain: new directions in research exploring the relation between cities and mood–anxiety disorders. *Depression and Anxiety,* 29, 186–201.

Gargett, R. H. 1999. Middle Palaeolithic burial is not a dead issue: the view from Qafzeh, Saint-Césaire, Kebara, Amud, and Dederiyeh. *Journal of Human Evolution,* 37, 27–90.

Garrett, L. 1994. *The Coming Plague: Newly Emerging Diseases in a World Out of Balance,* New York, NY: Farrar Straus and Giroux.

Gauthier Clerc, M., Lebarbenchon, C., and Thomas, F. 2007. Recent expansion of highly pathogenic avian influenza H5N1: a critical review. *Ibis,* 149, 202–14.

Geisbert, T. W., Bausch, D. G., and Feldmann, H. 2010. Prospects for immunisation against Marburg and Ebola viruses. *Reviews in Medical Virology,* 20, 344–57.

Goebel, T., Waters, M. R., and O'Rourke, D. H. 2008. The Late Pleistocene Dispersal of Modern Humans in the Americas. *Science,* 319, 1497–502.

Goldsworthy, P. D. and MacFarlane, A. C. 2002. Howard Florey, Alexander Fleming, and the Fairy Tale of Penicillin. *Medical Journal of Australia,* 176, 176–8.

Goodman, A. H. and Armelagos, G. J. 1988. Childhood Stress, Cultural Buffering, and Decreased Longevity in Prehistoric Populations. *American Anthropologist,* 90, 936–44.

Gootz, T. D. 2010. The Global Problem of Antibiotic Resistance. *Critical Reviews in Immunology,* 30, 79–93.

Green, A., Niels, C. H., and Pramming, S. K. 2002. The Changing World Demography of Type II Diabetes. *Diabetes/Metabolism Research and Reviews,* 19, 3–7.

Gregor, M. 2007. The Human/Animal Interface: Emergence and Resurgence of Zoonotic Infectious Diseases. *Critical Reviews in Microbiology,* 33, 243–99.

Gross, J. S., Neufeld, R. R., Libow, L. S., Gerber, I., and Rodstein, M. 1988. Autopsy Study of the Elderly Institutionalized Patient: Review of 234 Autopsies. *Archives of Internal Medicine,* 148, 173–6.

Guenther, M. 2007. Current Issues and Future Directions in Hunter-Gatherer Studies. *Anthropos,* 102, 371–88.

Gurven, M. and Kaplan, H. 2007. Longevity among hunter-gatherers: A cross-cultural examination. *Population and Development Review,* 33, 321–65.

Hales, C. N. and Barker, D. J. 2001. The thrifty phenotype hypothesis: type 2 diabetes. *British Medical Bulletin,* 60, 5–20.

Halliday, S. 1999. The Great Stink of London: Sir Joseph Bazalgette and the Cleansing of the Victorian Metropolis. Phoenix Mill, NY: Sutton.

Hansen, G. A. and Looft, C. 1895. Leprosy: in its clinical and pathological aspects. *The American Journal of the Medical Sciences,* 110, 586.

Harlan, J. 1971. Agricultural origins: centers and noncenters. *Science,* 174, 468–74.

Harn, A. D. 1978. Mississippian Settlement Patterns in the Central Illinois Valley. *In:* Smith, B. D. (ed.) *Mississippian Settlement Patterns,* New York, NY: Academic Press.

Harper, K. N., Ocampo, P. S., Steiner, B. M., George, R. W., Silverman, M. S., Boltin, S., Pillay, A., Saunders, N. J., and Armelagos, G. J. 2008. On the Origin of the Treponematoses: A Phylogenetic Approach. PLoS Neglected Tropical Diseases, 2 (1):e148, <http://www.plosntds.org/article/info%3Adoi%2F10.1371%2Fjournal.pntd.0000148>, last accessed March 30, 2013.

Harper, K. N., Zuckerman, M. K., Harper, M. L., Kingston, J., and Armelagos, G. J. 2011. The Origin and Antiquity of Syphilis Revisited: An Appraisal of Old World Pre-Columbian Evidence for Treponemal Infection. *American Journal of Physical Anthropology,* 146 (S53): 99–133.

Harper, K. N., Zuckerman, M. K., Turner, B. L., and Armelagos, G. J. In Press. Primates, Pathogens, and Evolution: A Context for Understanding Emerging Disease. *In:* Brinkworth, J. and Pechenkina, E. (eds) *Primates, Pathogens and Evolution,* New York, NY: Springer Publishing.

Hauspie, R. C., Vercauteran, M. and Susanne, C. 1997. Secular Changes in Growth and Maturation: An Update. *Acta Paediatrica,* 86, 20-7.

Hawkes, K. and O'Connell, J. F. 1992. On Optimal Foraging Models and Subsistence Transitions. *Current Anthropology,* 33, 63-6.

Henderson, D. A. 1980. Smallpox Eradication. *Public Health Reports,* 95, 422-6.

Hill, K. R. and Hurtado, A. M. 1996. *Ache Life History: The Ecology and Demography of a Foraging People,* Hawthorne, Aldine de Gruyter.

Hobbes, T. 1651. *Leviathan, or, The Matter, Forme, & Power of a Common-Wealth Ecclesiasticall and Civil,* London, Printer for A. Ckooke.

Hoffman, C. L. 1986. *The Punan: Hunters and Gatherers of Borneo,* Ann Arbor, MI: UMI Research Press.

Hopkins, D. 2002. *The Greatest Killer: Smallpox in History,* Chicago, IL: University of Chicago Press.

Hsu, E. 2006. Reflections on the "Discovery" of the Antimalarial Qinghao. *British Journal of Clinical Pharmacology,* 61, 666-70.

Hsu, E. and Barrett, R. 2009. Traditional Asian Medical Systems. *In:* Heggenhougan, K. (ed.) *International Encyclopedia of Public Health,* Oxford: Elsevier.

Huang, J., Yu, J., Hu, D., Wu, Y., Lu, J., Li, Y., Huang, Y., Azen, S. P., Dustin, L. D., and Detrano, R. C. 2010. The Farther From Town the Lower the Blood Pressure: Report From Rural Yunnan Province. *American Journal of Hypertension,* 24, 335-9.

Hunt, C. J. and Hunt, C. J. I. 2000. *Charles Hunt's Diet Evolution,* Beverly Hills, CA: Maximum Human Potential Productions.

Ingold, T. 1999. On the Social Relations of the Hunter-Gatherer Band. *In:* Lee, R. B. and Daly, R. (eds) *The Cambridge Encyclopedia of Hunter-Gatherers,* Cambridge UK: Cambridge University Press.

Ito, T., Kida, H., and Kawaoka, Y. 1996. Receptors of influenza A viruses: Implications for the role of pigs for the generation of pandemic human influenza viruses. In: Brown, L. E., Hampson, A. W. and Webster, R. G. (eds) *Options for the Control of Influenza III,* Amsterdam: Elsevier.

Jalland, P. 1996. *Death in the Victorian family,* Oxford: Oxford University Press.

Jemal, A., Bray, F., Center, M. M., Ferlay, J., Ward, E., and Forman, D. 2011. Global Cancer Statistics. *CA Cancer Journal for Clinicians,* 61, 69-90.

Jenike, M. 2001. Nutritional Ecology, Diet, Physical Activity, and Body Size. *In:* Panter-Brick, C., Layton, R. and Rowley-Conwy, P. (eds) *Hunter-Gatherers: An Interdisciplinary Perspective,* Cambridge UK: Cambridge University Press.

Jenner, E. 1798/2010. *The Three Original Papers on Vaccination against Smallpox,* London: Kessinger Publishing.

Johns, T. 1996. *The Origins of Human Diet and Medicine: Chemical Ecology,* Tuscon, AZ: University of Arizona Press.

Johnson, S. 2006. *The Ghost Map: The Story of London's Most Terrifying Epidemic - and How it Changed Science, Cities, and the Modern World,* New York, NY: Riverhead Books.

Jones, D. S. 2003. Virgin Soils Revisited. *The William and Mary Quarterly,* 60, 703–42.

Jones, K. E., Patel, N. G., Levy, M. A., Storeygard, A., Balk, D., Gittleman, J. L., and Daszak, P. 2008. Global trends in emerging infectious diseases. *Nature,* 451, 990–3.

Jones, W. P., Cin, Y.-W., and Kinghorn, A. D. 2006. The Role of Pharmacognosy in Modern Medicine and Pharmacy. *Current Drug Targets,* 7, 247–64.

Kanavos, P. 2006. The Rising Burden of Cancer in the Developing World. *Annals of Oncology,* 17, 815–23.

Kaplan, D. 2000. The Darker Side of the "Original Affluent Society." *Journal of Anthropological Research,* 56, 301–24.

Kelly, R. L. 1995. *The Foraging Spectrum: Diversity in Hunter-Gatherer Lifeways,* Washington DC: Smithsonian Institution Press.

Kennedy, K. 1984. Growth, nutrition and pathology in changing paleodemographic settings in South Asia. *In:* Cohen, M. N. and Armelagos, G. J. (eds) *Paleopathology at the Origins of Agriculture,* Orlando, FL: Academic Press.

Kim, J. Y., Shakow, A., Mate, K., Vanderwarker, C., Gupta, R., and Farmer, P. 2005. Limited good and limited vision: multidrug-resistant tuberculosis and global health policy. *Social Science and Medicine,* 61, 847–59.

Kinsella, K. and Velkoff, V. A. 2001. *An Aging World: 2001,* Washington DC: US Census Bureau.

Klebs, A. C. 1913. The Historic Evolution of Variolation. *Bulletin of the Johns Hopkins Hospital,* 24, 69–83.

Kleinman, A. M., Bloom, B. R., Saich, A., Mason, K. A., Aulino, F. 2008. Avian and Pandemic Influenza: A Biosocial Approach. *Journal of Infectious Diseases,* 197(S1): S1–3.

Kleinman, A. M. and Watson, J. L. (eds) 2006. *SARS in China: Prelude to a Pandemic?* Stanford, CA: Stanford University Press.

Kliks, M. M. 1990. Helminths as Heirlooms and Souvenirs: A Review of New World of Paleoparasitology. *Parasitology Today,* 6, 93–100.

Kolbert, E. 2009. The Flesh of Our Flesh. *The New Yorker.* New York, NY: Condé Nast.

Kopf, E. W. 1916. Florence Nightingale as Statistician. *Publications of the American Statistical Association,* 15, 388–404.

Kramer, M. S. 1998. Maternal nutrition, pregnancy outcome and public health policy. *Canadian Medical Association Journal,* 159, 663–5.

Kramer, M. S., McLean, F. H., Eason, E. L., and Usher, R. H. 1992. Maternal nutrition and spontaneous preterm birth. *American Journal of Epidemiology,* 136, 574–83.

Kudzma, E. C. 2006. Florence Nightingale and healthcare reform. *Nursing Science Quarterly,* 19(1) 61–4.

Kunitz, S. J. 1991. The Personal Physician and the Decline of Mortality. *In:* Schofield, R., Reher, D. and Bideau, A. (eds) *The Decline of Mortality in Europe,* Oxford: Oxford University Press.

Kuzawa, C. W. and Quinn, E. A. 2009. Developmental Origins of Adult Function and Health: Evolutionary Hypotheses. *Annual Review of Anthropology,* 38, 131–47.

Lamarre, J. M., Locke, J. B., Shaw, K. J., and Mankin, A. S. 2011. Low Fitness Cost of the Multidrug Resistance Gene cfr. *Antimicrobial Agents and Chemotherapy,* 55, 3714–19.

Lau, S. K. P., Woo, P. C. Y., Li, K. S. M., Huang, Y., Tsoi, H. W., Wong, B. H. L., Wong, S. S. Y., Leung, S. Y., Chan, K. H., and Yuen, K. Y. 2005. Severe acute respiratory syndrome coronavirus-like virus in Chinese horseshoe bats. *Proceedings of the National Academy of Sciences of the United States of America,* 102, 14040–5.

Lederburg, J., Shope, R. E., and Oaks, S. C. 1992. *Emerging Infections: Microbial Threats to Health in the United States,* Washington, DC: Institute of Medicine, National Academy Press.

Lee, R. B. 1990. *The !Kung San: Men, Women, and Work in a Foraging Society,* Cambridge UK, Cambridge University Press.

Lee, R. B. and Daly, R. 1999. Foragers and Others. *In:* Lee, R. B. and Daly, R. (eds) *The Cambridge Encyclopedia of Hunter-Gatherers,* Cambridge UK: Cambridge University Press.

Lee, R. B. and Devore, I. 1969. *Man the Hunter,* Chicago, IL: Aldine Publishing Company.

Lee, S., Chan, L. Y. Y., Chau, A. M. Y., Kwok, K. P. S., and Kleinman, A. 2005. The Experience of SARS-related Stigma at Amoy Gardens. *Social Science and Medicine,* 61, 2038–46.

Levy, S. B. 2002. *The Antibiotic Paradox: How Miracle Drugs Are Destroying the Miracle,* New York, NY: Plenum Press.

Lilienfeld, R. M. and Rathje, W. L. 1998. *Use Less Stuff: Environmentalism for Who We Really Are.* New York, NY: Ballantine Publishing Group.

Livi-Bacci, M. 2012. *A Concise History of World Population,* West Sussex, John Wiley and Sons.

Luangtongkum, T., Jeon, B., Han, J., Plummer, P., Logue, C. M., and Zhang, Q. 2009. Antibiotic resistance in Campylobacter: emergence, transmission and persistence. *Future Microbiology,* 4, 189–200.

MacNeish, R. S. 1992. *The Origins of Agriculture and Settled Life,* Norman, OK: University of Oklahoma Press.

MacPherson, D. W., Gushulak, B. D., Baine, W. B., Bala, S., Gubbins, P. O., Holtom, P., and Segarra Newham, M. 2009. Population Mobility, Globalization, and Antimicrobial Drug Resistance. *Emerging Infectious Diseases,* 15, 1727–32.

Markel, H. 2003. *When Germs Travel: Six Major Epidemics That Have Invaded America and the Fears They Have Unleashed,* New York, Vintage Books.

Markel, H., Navarro, J., Sloan, A., Michelson, J., Am, S., and Cetron, M. 2007. Nonpharmacological Interventions Implemented by U.S. Cities During the 1918–1919 Influenza Pandemic. *Journal of the American Medical Association,* 298, 644–54.

Marlowe, F. W. 2005. Hunter-Gatherers and Human Evolution. *Evolutionary Anthropology,* 14, 54–67.

Marshall, B. M. and Levy, S. B. 2011. Food Animals and Antimicrobials: Impacts on Human Health. *Clinical Microbiology Reviews,* 24, 718–33.

Martin, D. L., Armelagos, G. J., Goodman, A. H., and Van Gerven, D.P. 1984. The Effects of Socioeconomic change in Prehistoric Africa: Sudanese Nubia as a Case Study. *In:* Cohen, M.N. and Armelagos, G.J. (eds) *Paleopathology at the Origins of Agriculture,* Orlando, FL: Academic Press.

Mayer-Foulkes, D. 2001. "Convergence Clubs in Cross-Country Life Expectancy Dynamics." Helsinki: United Nations University–World Institute for Development Economics Research. Discussion Paper No. 2001/134.

Mays, S., Brickley, M., and Ives, R. 2006. Skeletal Manifestations of Rickets in Infants and Young Children in a Historic Population from England. *American Journal of Physical Anthropology,* 129, 362–74.

McDonald, L. 2001. Florence Nightingale and the Early Origins of Evidence-Based Nursing. *Evidence Based Nursing,* 4, 68–9.

McGee, G. 2007. Thanks, Andrew Speaker. *The Scientist,* 21, 121–3.

McGillicuddy, T. J. 1898. Tuberculosis: Its Seed, Its Soil, and Its Treatment by Medical Sepsis. *Journal of the American Medical Association,* 30, 1395–7.

McKeown, T. 1965. Medicine and World Population. *Journal of Chronic Disease,* 18, 1067–77.

McKeown, T. 1976. *The Modern Rise of Population,* New York, NY: Academic Press.

McKeown, T. 1988. *The Origins of Human Disease,* Oxford: Basil Blackwell.

McKeown, T., Brown, R. G., and Record, R. G. 1972. An Interpretation of the Modern Rise in Population in Europe. *Population Studies,* 26, 345–82.

McKinney, K. R., Gong, Y. Y., and Lewis, T. G. 2006. Environmental transmission of SARS at Amoy Gardens. *Journal of Environmental Health,* 68, 26–30.

McNeill, W. H. 1976. *Plagues and Peoples,* Garden City, Anchor/Doubleday.

Mead, P. S., Slutsker, L., Dietz, V., Mccaig, L. F., Bresee, J. S., Shapiro, C., Griffin, P. M., and Tauxe, R. V. 1999. Food-related Illness and Death in the United States. *Emerging Infectious Diseases,* 5, 607–25.

Mercer, T. J. 1985. Smallpox and Epidemiological-Demographic Change in Europe: The Role of Vaccination. *Population Studies,* 39, 287–307.

Meyer, R. D. 1983. Legionella Infections—A Review of Five Years of Research. *Reviews of Infectious Diseases,* 5, 258–78.

Morgan, A. 2006. Avian influenza: An agricultural perspective. *Journal of Infectious Diseases*, 194, S139–46.

Morrow, P. A. 1904. *Social Diseases and Marriage: Social Prophylaxis*, New York, NY: Lea Brothers Company.

Mugusi, F., Swai, A. B. M., Alberti, K. G. M., and Mclarty, D. G. 1990. Increased Prevalence of Diabetes-Mellitus in Patients with Pulmonary Tuberculosis in Tanzania. *Tubercle*, 71, 271–6.

Munro, N. D. and Grosman, L. 2010. Early evidence (ca. 12,000 B.P.) for feasting at a burial cave in Israel. *Proceedings of the National Academy of Sciences*, 107, 15362–6.

Neel, J. V. 1982. The Thrifty Genotype Revisited. *In:* Kobberling, J., and Tattersall, R. (ed.) *Genetics of Diabetes Mellitus*, Academic Press: London.

Nelson, M., Hochberg, J., Dinardo, A., and Armelagos, G. J. 2010. Spectroscopic Characterization of Tetracycline in Skeletal Remains of an Ancient Population from Sudanese Nubia, 350CE–550CE. *American Journal of Physical Anthropology*, 143, 151–4.

Nichter, M. 2008. *Global Health: Why Cultural Perceptions, Social Representations, and Biopolitics Matter*, Tuscon, AZ: University of Arizona Press.

Nightingale, F. 1859/1992. *Notes on nursing: What it is, and what it is not*, Philadelphia, PA: Lippincott Williams and Wilkins.

Normark, B. H. and Normark, S. 2002. Evolution and Spread of Antibiotic Resistance. *Journal of Internal Medicine*, 252, 91–106.

Noymer, A. and Garenne, M. 2000. The 1918 influenza epidemic's effects on sex differentials in mortality in the United States. *Population and Development Review*, 26, 565–81.

Ó Gráda, C. 2009. *Famine: A Short History*, Princeton, NJ: Princeton University Press.

Olsen, B., Munster, V. J., Wallensten, A., Waldenstrom, J., Osterhaus, A., and Fouchier, R. A. M. 2006. Global patterns of influenza A virus in wild birds. *Science*, 312, 384–8.

Omran, A. R. 1971. The epidemiologic transition: A theory of the epidemiology of population change. *Millbank Memorial Fund Quarterly*, 49, 509–38.

Patz, J. A., Epstein, P. R., Burke, T. A., and Balbous, J. M. 1996. Global Climate Change and Emerging Infectious Diseases. *JAMA*, 275, 217–23.

Paynter, R. and Mcguire, R. (eds) 1991. *The Archaeology of Inequality*, Oxford: Basil Blackwell.

Pennington, R. 2001. Hunter-Gatherer Demography. *In:* Panter-Brick, C., Layton, R. and Rowley-Conwy, P. (eds) *Hunter-Gatherers: An Interdisciplinary Perspective*, Cambridge, UK: Cambridge University Press.

Perri, A. 2008. The Quarantine Conundrum. *The Meducator*, 1, <http://digitalcommons. mcmaster.ca/meducator/vol1/iss12/10>, last accessed March 30, 2013.

Petersdorf, R. G. 1986. Training, Cost Containment, and Practice: Effect on Infectious Diseases. *Review of Infectious Diseases*, 8, 478–87.

Piepenbrink, H., Herrmann, B., and Hoffmann, P. 1983. Tetracycline-Like Flourescences in Buried Human Bones. *Zeitschrift Fur Rechtsmedizin-Journal of Legal Medicine,* 91, 71–4.

Piperno, D. R. 2001. On Maize and the Sunflower. *Science,* 292, 2260–1.

Plotkin, S. A. 2005. Vaccines: Past, Present, and Future. *Nature Medicine Supplement,* 11, S5–11.

Ponce-De-Leon, A., Garcia-Garcia, M. D., Garcia-Sancho, C., Gomez-Perez, F. J., Valdespino-Gomez, J. L., Olaiz-Fernandez, G., Rojas, R., Ferreyra-Reyes, L., Cano-Arellano, B., Bobadilla, M., Small, P. M., and Sifuentes-Osornio, J. 2004. Tuberculosis and diabetes in southern Mexico. *Diabetes Care,* 27, 1584–90.

Popkin, B. M. 1994. The Nutrition Transition in Low-Income Countries: An Emerging Crisis. *Nutrition Reviews,* 52, 285–98.

Preston, R. 1994. *The Hot Zone,* New York, NY: Random House.

Preston, S. H. 1980. Causes and Consequences of Mortality Declines in Less Developed Countries During the Twentieth Century. *Population and Economic Change in Developing Countries,* Chicago, IL: University of Chicago Press.

Price, T. D. and Gebauer, A. B. 1995. *Last Hunters, First Farmers: New Perspectives on the Prehistoric Transition to Agriculture,* Santa Fe, NM: School of American Research Press.

Quetel, C., Braddock, J., and Pike, B. 1990. *History of Syphilis,* Cambridge, Polity Press.

Quetelet, M. A. 1842. *A Treatise on Man,* Edinburgh, William and Robert Chambers.

Ramenofsky, A. F. 1987. *Vectors of Death: The Archaeology of European Contact,* Albuquerque, NM: University of New Mexico Press.

Rathburn, T. A. 1984. Skeletal Pathology from the Paleolithic through the Metal Ages in Iran and Iraq. *In:* Cohen, M. N. and Armelagos, G. J. (eds) *Paleopathology at the Origins of Agriculture,* Orlando, FL: Academic Press.

Reinhardt, A., Koehler, T., Wood, P., Rohner, P., Dumas, J.-L., Ricou, B., and Van Delden, C. 2007. Development and persistence of antimicrobial resistance in *Pseudomonas aeruginosa*: a longitudinal observation in mechanically ventilated patients. *Antimicrobial Agents and Chemotherapy,* 51, 1341–50.

Reitsema, L. J. and Vercellotti, G. 2012. Stable Isotope Evidence for Sex- and Status-Based Variations in Diet and Life History at Medieval Trino Vercellese, Italy. *American Journal of Physical Anthropology,* 148(4): 589–600.

Riley, J. C. 2005. The Timing and Pace of Health Transitions Around the World. *Population and Development Review,* 31, 741–64.

Rios, J. L. and Recio, M. C. 2005. Medicinal Plants and Antimicrobial Activity. *Journal of Ethnopharmacology,* 100, 80–4.

Rolls, B. J., Rolls, E. T., and Rowe, E. A. 1982. The Influence of Variety on Human Food Selection and Intake. *In:* Baker, L. M. (ed.) *The Psychobiology of Food Selection,* Westport, CT: AVI.

Root, H. F. 1934. The Association of Diabetes and Tuberculosis. *New England Journal of Medicine,* 210, 1–13.

Rouchoux, J. A. 1834. *Dictionnaire de Médecine, Vol, VIII,* Paris.

Rousseau, J. J. 1754. *A Discourse on a Subject Proposed by the Academy of Dijon: What is the Origin of Inequality among Men, and is it Authorized by Natural Law?* Translated by G. D. H. Cole, public domain. Rendered into HTML and text by Jon Roland of the Constitution Society. <http://www.constitution.org/jjr/ineq.htm>, last accessed October 31, 2001.

Ruprecht, K., Mayer, J., Sauter, M., Roemer, K., and Mueller-Lantzsch, N. 2008. Endogenous retroviruses. *Cellular and Molecular Life Sciences,* 65, 3366–82.

Ryan, F. P. 2004. Human Endogenous Retroviruses: A Symbiotic Perspective. *Journal of the Royal Society of Medicine,* 97, 560–5.

Sachs, J. S. 2007. *Good Germs, Bad Germs: Health and Survival in a Bacterial World,* New York, NY: Hill and Wang.

Sack, D. A., Sack, R. B., Nair, G. B., and Siddique, A. K. 2004. Cholera. *Lancet,* 363, 223–33.

Sahlins, M. 1968. Notes on the Original Affluent Society. *In:* Lee, R.B. and DeVore, I. (eds) *Man the Hunter,* New York, NY: Aldine.

Saker, L., Lee, K., Cannito, B., Gilmore, A., and Campbell-Lendrum, D. 2004. *Globalization and Infectious Diseases: A Review of the Linkages,* Geneva: UNICEF/UNDP/World Bank/ WHO Special Program for Research and Training in Tropical Diseases.

Salamini, F., Ozkan, H., Brandolini, A., Schafer-Pregl, R., and Martin, W. 2002. Genetics and geography of wild cereal domestication in the Near East. *Nature Reviews Genetics,* 3, 429–41.

Salomon, J. A. and Murray, C. J. L. 2002. The Epidemiological Transition Revisited: Compositional Models by Age and Sex. *Population and Development Review,* 28, 205–28.

Satcher, D. 1995. Emerging Infections: Getting Ahead of the Curve. *Emerging Infectious Diseases,* 1 (1): 1–6.

Schaible, U. E. and Kaufman, S. H. E. 2007. Malnutrition and Infection: Complex Mechanisms and Global Impacts. *PLoS Medicine,* 4, 806–11.

Schurr, T. G. 2004. The Peopling of the New World: Perspectives from Molecular Anthropology. *Annual Review of Anthropology,* 33, 551–83.

Sethi, S. 2002. Bacterial pneumonia—Managing a deadly complication of influenza in older adults with comorbid disease. *Geriatrics,* 57, 56–61.

Sherertz, R. J., Reagan, D. R., Hampton, K. D., Robertson, K. L., Streed, S. A., Hoen, H. M., Thomas, R., and Gwaltney, J. M. 1996. A cloud adult: The *Staphylococcus aureus*—Virus interaction revisited. *Annals of Internal Medicine,* 124, 539–47.

Singer, M. and Clair, S. 2003. Syndemics and Public Health: Reconceptualizing Disease in Bio-Social Context. *Medical Anthropology Quarterly,* 17, 423–41.

Smith, P. 1984. Archaeological and Skeletal Evidence for Dietary Change During the Late Pliestocene/Early Holocene in the Levant. *In:* Cohen, M. N. and Armelagos, G. J. (eds) *Paleopathology at the Origins of Agriculture*, Orlando, FL: Academic Press.

Smith, P. W., Seip, C. W., Schaefer, S. C., and Bell-Dixon, C. 2000. Microbiologic survey of long-term care facilities. *American Journal of Infection Control*, 28, 8–13.

Smith, V. H., Jones II, T. P., and Smith, M. 2005. Host Nutrition and Infectious Disease: An Ecological View. *Frontiers in Ecology and the Environment*, 3, 268–74.

Snow, J. 1855. *On the Mode of Communication of Cholera*, London: John Churchill.

Soares, R. R. 2007. On the Determinants of Mortality Reductions in the Developing World. *Population and Development Review*, 33, 247–87.

Solecki, R. S. 1971. Shanidar: The First Flower People. *Science*, 190, 880–1.

Sommer, J. D. 1999. The Shanidar IV "Flower Burial": a Re-evaluation of Neanderthal Burial Ritual. *Cambridge Archaeological Journal*, 9, 127–9.

Speller, C. F., Kemp, B. M., Wyatt, S. D., Monroe, C., Lipe, W. D., Arndt, U. M., and Yang, D. Y. 2010. Ancient mitochondrial DNA analysis reveals complexity of indigenous North American turkey domestication. *Proceedings of the National Academy of Sciences of the United States of America*, 107, 2807–12.

Sprent, J. F. A. 1969. Evolutionary aspects of immunity of zooparasitic infections. *In:* Jackson, G. J. (ed.) *Immunity to Parasitic Animals*, New York: Appleton.

Stiner, M. C., Munro, N. D., Surovell, T. A., Tchernov, E., and Bar-Yosef, O. 1999. Paleolithic Population Growth Pulses Evidenced by Small Animal Exploitation. *Science*, 283, 190–4.

Stuart-Macadam, P. 1987. Porotic Hyperostosis: New Evidence to Support the Anemia Theory. *American Journal of Physical Anthropology*, 74, 521–6.

Stuart-Macadam, P. 1989. Nutritional Deficiency Disease: A Survey of Scurvy, Rickets, and Iron Deficiency Anemia *In*: Iscan, M. Y. and Kennedy, K. (eds) *Reconstruction of Life from the Skeleton*, New York, NY: Wiley-Liss.

Tanner, J. M. 1987. Growth as a Mirror of the Condition of Society: Secular Trends and Class Distinctions. *Acta Paediatrica Japonica*, 29, 96–103.

Tanner, J. M. 1992. Growth as a Measure of the Nutritional and Hygienic Status of a Population. *Hormone Research*, 38, 108–15.

Tauxe, R. V., Mintz, E. D., and Quick, R. E. 1995. Epidemic Cholera in the New World: Translating Field Epidemiology into New Prevention Strategies. *Emerging Infectious Diseases*, 1, 141–6.

Thompson, K. M. and Tebbens, R. J. 2006. Retrospective Cost Analyses for Polio Vaccination in the United States. *Risk Analysis*, 26, 1423–40.

Thompson, W. W., Comanor, L., and Shay, D. K. 2006. Epidemiology of seasonal influenza: Use of surveillance data and statistical models to estimate the burden of disease. *Journal of Infectious Diseases*, 194, S82–91.

Turnbaugh, P. J., Quince, C., Faith, J. J., McHardy, A. C., Yatsunenko, T., Niazi, F., Affourtit, J., Egholm, M., Henrissat, B., Knight, R., and Gordon, J. I. 2010. Organismal, genetic, and transcriptional variation in the deeply sequenced gut microbiomes of identical twins. *Proceedings of the National Academy of Sciences of the United States of America*, 107, 7503–8.

Ullrey, D. E. 2005. Nutrition and Predisposition to Infectious Disease. *Journal of Zoo and Wildlife Medicine*, 24, 304–14.

Ursell, L. K., Clemente, J. C., Rideout, J. R., Gevers, D., Caporaso, J. G., and Knight, R. 2012. The interpersonal and intrapersonal diversity of human-associated microbiota in key body sites. *Journal of Allergy and Clinical Immunology*, 129, 1204–8.

Vallin, J. 1991. Mortality in Europe from 1720 to 1914: Long-Term Trends and Changes in Patterns by Age and Sex. *In:* Schofield, R., Reher, D. and Bideau, A. (eds) *The Decline of Mortality in Europe*, Oxford: Oxford University Press.

Van Der Linde, D., Konings, E. E. M., Slager, M. A., Witsenburg, M., Helbing, W. A., Takkenberg, J. J. M., and Roos-Hesselink, J. W. 2011. Birth Prevalence of Congenital Heart Disease Worldwide: A Systematic Review and Meta-Analysis. *Journal of the American College of Cardiology*, 58, 2241–7.

Van Gerven, D., Hummert, J., Pendergast Moore, K., and Sanford, M. K. 1990. Nutrition, Disease, and the Human Life Cycle: A Bioethnography of a Medieval Nubian Community. *In:* Derousseau, C. J. (ed.) *Primate Life History and Evolution*, New York: Wiley-Liss.

Varro, M. T. 1783/1934. On Agriculture, Book 1. *In:* Hooper, W. D. and Ash, H. B. (eds) *Cato and Varro on Agriculture, Loeb Classical Library, Number* 283, <http://penelope.uchicago.edu/Thayer/E/Roman/Texts/Varro/de_Re_Rustica/1*.html#12.2>, last accessed March 30, 2013. Cambridge: Loeb Classical Library, Harvard University Press.

Vince, G. 2011. An Epoch Debate. *Science,* 334, 32–7.

Walkowitz, J. R. 1982. *Prostitution and Victorian society: Women, Class, and the State,* Cambridge: Cambridge University Press.

Wapler, U., Crubezy, E., and Schultz, M. 2004. Is cribra orbitalia synonymous with anemia? Analysis and interpretation of cranial pathology in Sudan. *American Journal of Physical Anthropology*, 123, 333–9.

Waters, M. R. and Stafford, T. W. J. 2007. Redefining the Age of Clovis: Implications for the Peopling of the Americas. *Science,* 315, 1122–6.

Watts, I. 1715. *Divine Songs attempted in Easy Language for the Use of Children with some Additional Compusures*, London, M. Lawrence. Reprinted and sold by B. Franklin and D. Hall, 1750; facsimile, London: Oxford University Press, 1971. <http://www.english.uga.edu/wblake/SONGS/hymns/watts.html>, last accessed March 30 2013.

Watts, S. 1997. *Epidemics and History: Disease, Power, and Imperialism,* New Haven, CT: Yale University Press.

Weiss, R. A. 2001. Animal origins of human infectious disease. *Philosophical Transactions of the Royal Society of London, Series B-Biological Sciences,* 356, 957–77.

Wiener, P. and Wilkinson, S. 2011. Deciphering the genetic basis of animal domestication. *Proceedings of the Royal Society, Series B-Biological Sciences,* 278, 3161–70.

Winau, F., Westphal, O., and Winau, R. 2004. Paul Ehrlich—in search of the magic bullet. *Microbes and Infection,* 6, 786–9.

Winterhalder, B. 2001. The Behavioral Ecology of Hunter-Gatherers. *In:* Panter-Brick, C., Layton, R. and Rowley-Conwy, P. (eds) *Hunter-Gatherers: An Interdisciplinary Perspective,* Cambridge, UK: Cambridge University Press.

Wolfe, N. D. 2011. *Viral Storm: The Dawn of a New Pandemic,* New York, NY: Henry Holt and Company.

Wolfe, N. D., Daszak, P., Kilpatrick, A. M., and Burke, D. S. 2005. Bushmeat hunting, deforestation, and prediction of zoonoses emergence. *Emerging Infectious Diseases,* 11, 1822–7.

Wolfe, N. D., Dunavan, C. P., and Diamond, J. 2007. Origins of major human infectious diseases. *Nature,* 447, 279–83.

Wolfe, N. D., Switzer, W. M., Carr, J. K., Bhullar, V. B., Shanmugam, V., Tamoufe, U., Prosser, A. T., Torimiro, J. N., Wright, A., Mpoudi-Ngole, E., Mccutchan, F. E., Birx, D. L., Folks, T. M., Burke, D. S., and Heneine, W. 2004. Naturally acquired simian retrovirus infections in central African hunters. *Lancet,* 363, 932–7.

Wolfe, R. J. 1982. Alaska's great sickness, 1900: an epidemic of measles and influenza in a virgin soil population. *Proceedings of the American Philosophical Society,* 126, 91–121.

Wong, S. S. Y. and Yuen, K. 2006. Avian influenza virus infections in humans. *Chest,* 129, 156–68.

Wood, J. W., Milner, G. R., Harpending, H. C., and Weiss, K. M. 1992. The Osteological Paradox. *Current Anthropology,* 33, 343–70.

Woods, R. 1991. Public Health and Public Hygiene: The Urban Environment in the Late Nineteenth and Early Twentieth Centuries. *In:* Schofield, R., Reher, D., and Bideau, A. (eds) *The Decline of Mortality in Europe,* Oxford: Oxford University Press.

Woolhouse, M. and Gaunt, E. 2007. Ecological Origins of Novel Human Pathogens. *Critical Reviews of Microbiology,* 33, 231–42.

World Health Organization 2007. *How to Improve the Use of Medicines by Consumers,* Geneva: World Health Organization.

World Health Organization 2010a. *Guidelines for the Treatment of Malaria,* Geneva: World Health Organization.

World Health Organization 2010b. *Multidrug and Extensively Drug-Resistant TB (M/XDR-TB): 2010 Global Report on Surveillance and Response.* Geneva: World Health Organization.

World Resources 1996–97 1996. *A Guide to the Global Environment: The Urban Environment,* Washington, DC: World Resources International.

Wright, A., Zignol, M., Van Deun, A., Falzon, D., Gerdes, S. R., Feldman, K., Hoffner, S., Drobniewski, F., Barrera, L., Van Soolingen, D., Boulabhal, F., Paramasivan, C. N., Kam, K. M., Mitarai, S., Nunn, P., Raviglione, M., and Global Project Anti, T. B. D. R. 2009. Epidemiology of antituberculosis drug resistance 2002–07: an updated analysis of the Global Project on Anti-Tuberculosis Drug Resistance Surveillance. *Lancet,* 373, 1861–73.

Wrigley, E. A., Davies, R. S., Oeppen, J. A., and Scofield, R. S. 1997. *English Population History from Family Reconstitution,* 1580–1837, Cambridge: Cambridge University Press.

Yajnik, C. S. 2004. Early Life Origins of Insulin Resistance and Type 2 Diabetes in India and Other Asian Countries. *Journal of Nutrition,* 134, 205–10.

Yersin, A. 1894. La Peste Bubonique à Hong Kong. *Annales de lInstitut Pasteur,* 8, 662–7.

Zedong, M. 1958. Farewell to the God of Plague. *Poems: Selected Works of Mao Tse-tung.* <http://www.marxists.org/reference/archive/mao/selected-works/poems/poems25.htm> last accessed March 30, 2013.

Zhu, T., Korber, B. T., Nahmias, A. J., Hooper, E., Sharp, P. M., and Ho, D. D. 1998. An African HIV-1 sequence from 1959 and implications for the origin of the epidemic. *Nature,* 391, 594–7.

Index